To
America's
Health

*The Hoover Institution
gratefully acknowledges
the generous support of*

RATHMANN FAMILY FOUNDATION

WILLIAM J. RUTTER

*for substantially underwriting this
research project and publication.*

To America's Health

A Proposal to Reform the Food and Drug Administration

Henry I. Miller, MD

HOOVER INSTITUTION PRESS
Stanford University Stanford, California

Hoover Institution Press Publication No. 482

First printing, 2000
06   05   04   03   02   01   00   9 8 7 6 5 4 3 2 1

Manufactured in the United States of America
The paper used in this publication meets the minimum requirements
of American National Standard for Information Sciences—Permanence
of Paper for Printed Library Materials, ANSI Z39.48-1984. ⊗

Library of Congress Cataloging-in-Publication Data
Miller, Henry I.
   To America's health : a proposal to reform the Food and Drug
Administration / Henry I. Miller.
       p.   cm. — (Hoover Institution Press publication ; 482)
   Includes bibliographical references and index.
   ISBN 0-8179-9902-7 (pbk. : alk. paper)
   1. Pharmaceutical policy—United States.   2. United States. Food
and Drug Administration.   3. Drugs—Law and legislation—United
States.   4. Pharmaceutical industry—United States.   I. Title.
II. Series.
RA401.A3 M55   2000
353.9'98'0973—dc21   00-031937

In memory of my mother,

SADIE FELDMAN MILLER
(1910–1999),

*who taught me that with
perseverance and integrity
all things are possible.*

Contents

Figures

Foreword

Unfettered markets can sometimes harm competitors and the general public as well. Examples include companies that dump their waste indiscriminately, polluting the environment, and those that create monopolies to restrict competition and boost prices to consumers.

Government regulation is often designed to counter these market imperfections. For example, the Environmental Protection Agency's regulation of SO_2 emissions from coal-fired generating plants is designed to protect people from acid rain. Antitrust suits, such as the one brought by the Department of Justice against Microsoft, are designed to force industry giants to lower their prices and allow more competition. But regulations intended to improve on the performance of markets sometimes generate unintended or unexpected negative consequences. Consider, for instance, several cases involving natural resources. Restrictions on the ability of willing buyers and willing sellers of water to trade are having adverse impacts on salmon recovery in the Pacific Northwest. Environmentalists are often willing to pay to keep water in the stream for spawning habitat, but many states have laws that do not allow farmers to sell their water to these environmentalists. Another example is the Endangered Species Act, whose regulations are supposed to prevent people from "taking" species, a term interpreted to mean taking away their habitat. But regulations that prohibit landowners from harvesting timber if red-cockaded woodpeckers are found on their property have encouraged landowners to cut their timber before it gets old enough to attract woodpeckers—an example of a worthy goal thwarted by distorted regulatory incentives. Hence, in North Carolina landowners with no known red-cockaded woodpecker colonies in the vicinity let their trees grow until they are about sixty years old, whereas landowners with abundant nearby colonies of the birds cut trees for pulpwood when they are fifteen years old. Regulations on fishing are even more ridiculous. To prevent overharvesting of oysters, Maryland at one time institutionalized underproductivity by requiring that oyster dredges be towed behind sail-powered (as opposed to motor-powered) boats on all but two days of the week; this, of course, drastically limited the catch. Until recently the entire season for commercial halibut fishing in Alaska was two days. These measures might have helped to prevent overfishing, but they unnecessarily increased the costs of harvesting the catch.

Outside the natural resource arena, many other regulations are infamous for their unintended or costly consequences. Economists have documented damage to the airline and trucking industries from federal (nonsafety) regulations, which was reversed by deregulation. For example, before deregulation, intrastate moving rates, which were unregulated, were often nearly 50 percent less than (interstate) rates regulated by the Interstate Commerce Commission. The notoriously ineffective and expensive 1977 amendments to the Clean Air Act required power companies to install millions of dollars of equipment to scrub their emissions and increased the cost of electricity generation perhaps by as much $5 billion. But the air would have been cleaner and electricity costs lower if the companies had simply burned lower-sulphur coal. Thus, air pollution—what the new regulations were designed specifically to prevent—was exacerbated by inflexible "design" standards prescribed by government.

Fortunately, the average U.S. citizen is wealthy enough that these inefficiencies are barely perceived. Or, as I often quip, we are lucky we are so rich or we could not afford all these efficiencies. Because each inefficiency has costs that are trivial compared to our gross domestic product (GDP), and because the costs are commonly widely distributed, there is often little pressure for change. To make matters worse, certain interest groups that benefit from the regulations fight to get them and to keep them in place. In the case of the emissions potentially subject to the Clean Air Act, for example, older power plants were "grandfathered" into the legislation, which meant they were exempt from the regulations. Not surprisingly the operators of those plants supported the regulations because they raised costs to competitors, and Eastern, high-sulphur coal interests supported regulations that discouraged the use of Western, low-sulphur coal. Businesses that know how to comply with complex regulations also prefer them because they act as a market-entry barrier, keeping out new entrants who would have a steep learning curve (and possibly huge expenses) to negotiate the regulatory maze. Finally, the bureaucrats who oversee regulations are unlikely to lobby for deregulation if it would mean eliminating their own jobs, limiting their advancement, or reducing their perquisites. In short, efficiency has no constituency. Even when it does, the burden is on the reformer to show that the regulations are worse than a freer market would be.

Enter Henry Miller and this volume, *To America's Health: A Proposal to Reform the Food and Drug Administration.* Reformer Miller is taking on the regulation of new drugs, probably the most pervasive regulatory system in the United States, and one that affects every U.S. citizen. Since 1962, the Food and Drug Administration (FDA) has certified the safety and effectiveness of all new marketed drugs through a licensing procedure designed to protect consumers against harms that they could never anticipate. Who could deny that such harms occur, given the well-known accounts of pre-FDA "snake-oil" and post-FDA drugs withdrawn from the market because of dangerous side effects.

But again, the counterintuitive must be considered; namely, the FDA's current regulatory regime may actually make consumers worse off. As with other regulations, policy analysts have mustered abundant evidence to support such a hypothesis. Henry Miller marshals this evidence to argue that unnecessary delays in regulatory approval of new

drugs that result from the anxiety, timidity, or incompetence of regulators can be costly because such delays mean that people must forgo
potential benefits. In some cases this means that people will suffer or
die. In addition to these forgone health benefits, FDA regulations raise
the costs of drug research and development and, ultimately, the costs
of drugs to consumers. As these regulatory costs are becoming better
known and as health care costs impose a heavier burden on our society,
the pressure is building for policy reforms that will lower health care
costs without compromising safety. Regrettably, regulatory reform is
seldom high on the list of remedies.

As a medical doctor by training and a former federal regulator, Henry
Miller is aware of the benefits that accrue to society when unsuspecting
consumers are protected from inadequately tested, dangerous drugs.
Therefore, he rejects deregulation that would throw the baby out with
the bath water. He examines the data that show that the existing regulatory regime is broken and asks how it can be fixed. His conclusion,
bolstered by the work of many other scholars and studies, is that the
problem lies in the federal monopoly over drug regulation and the
absence of incentives to speed up the regulatory process in order to get
needed drugs to consumers. (In fact, he argues that the current system
has created incentives to do exactly the opposite.) Therefore his solution
is quite simple: establish private drug certifying bodies (DCBs) that
would contract with pharmaceutical companies to oversee the testing
and evaluation of their drugs and that would compete with one another.
This would lower the cost of the approval process while maintaining
product quality. Miller's proposal would not alter the current basic
requirement that marketed drugs be safe and effective, and it includes
a role for the FDA, making it the certifier of certifiers rather than a
certifier of products. Hence, the FDA would decide which companies
are qualified to act as DCBs and, by way of analogy, give a "Good
Housekeeping Seal of Approval."

Not everyone will like Dr. Miller's reform proposals. Libertarians will
think he does not go far enough to get the government out of health
care, and liberals will cavil that consumers need more protection and

government involvement, not less. But everyone should be convinced that the current system is broken and needs fixing. The reader of this book will also agree that Henry Miller has devised a coherent and scholarly reform proposal with which all serious policy analysts must reckon. If we choose to carry on with the status quo, we will face continually escalating costs with little benefit; if we wait for the perfect reform policy, perfection will be the enemy of the good. But if we follow Dr. Miller's prescription, we just might be on road to a policy reform that will actually give us more for less. Read on.

Terry L. Anderson
Senior Fellow, Hoover Institution
and Executive Director, Political Economy Research Center

Preface

The Food and Drug Administration (FDA) is the national gatekeeper for the introduction of new drugs and other products into U.S. markets. Its complex regulatory culture, which has evolved over almost a century, has seen the accretion of regulatory responsibilities and continually expanding organization. Now funded at approximately a billion dollars a year, with some ten thousand employees, the FDA regulates several major classes of consumer products—including human and animal drugs, medical devices, foods and cosmetics—worth more than $1 *trillion* annually.

The FDA's centralized evaluation of new drugs, performed by its own employees, differs in several ways from its counterparts in other modern industrialized nations, which rely heavily on experts from the private sector. (It should be noted that in either case, however, the data are generated by industry.) In these countries, regulatory agencies' review components are small compared to their FDA counterparts and regulatory decisions generally are met with much less public interest and media attention than the FDA receives. At the same time, such foreign systems for drug review and approval as the United Kingdom's Medicines Control Agency and the European Union's European Agency for the Evaluation of Medicinal Products can be viewed as more efficient than the FDA because they regularly perform reviews as or more rapidly with significantly less staff and expense.

Drug regulatory agencies in the United States and abroad have from time to time been criticized for slowness and inefficiency. The constitutional separation of executive and legislative responsibilities in the United States, however, makes significant regulatory reform more difficult to accomplish than in countries with a parliamentary form of government. During the mid-1980s, for example, when the British government was troubled by delays in its approval of new drugs, Prime Minister Margaret Thatcher established a small team to evaluate the slowness in product approvals and recommend improvements. The team rapidly conducted its study and produced a fifty-six-page typed report, and the prime minister quickly implemented the recommended sweeping organizational changes. The result was the establishment of a new Medicines Control Agency, self-funded by user fees from industry and designed to be run like an efficient private-sector service organization. The Medicines Control Agency today operates with a much smaller staff and budget than the FDA, although the agencies' functions, review times, and standards for approval are similar.

At about the same time as the United Kingdom was evaluating its drug review system, the United States, under the leadership of Vice President George Bush, also began a government study on ways to speed up the drug approval process. In contrast to the expeditiousness with which recommendations were made and implemented in the United Kingdom, however, in the United States the process consumed vastly greater resources, took longer, attracted substantial political attention, and resulted in only modest changes to the existing system of drug evaluation and approval. President Bush's executive branch reforms included the expansion of expedited, or fast-track, reviews to more classes of products than just the treatment of AIDS (which had previously been the case) and wider use of surrogate clinical markers as criteria for drug effectiveness.

The Bush administration's reforms of the drug approval process emanated from the President's Council on Competitiveness. One important question considered by the council was whether the drug approval process would be improved by the FDA's use of nongovernment experts to evaluate particular products. The council briefly considered the use of expert organizations analogous to Underwriters Laboratories, a model in some ways similar to that proposed by Henry Miller in this volume. To assess the feasibility of using nongovernment reviewers, the FDA agreed to establish a pilot program in which the agency would contract with nongovernmental experts to conduct certain routine reviews on a limited, experimental basis. When President Bush publicly announced these reforms, several leading congressional Democrats strongly condemned the FDA's limited contracting out of a few routine reviews. Their partisan resistance to this experimental pilot program illustrates how the political process in Washington can inhibit even the most modest reforms: A good-faith effort to increase a regulatory agency's productivity and available expertise through the use of outside experts was falsely represented as a change designed to permit pharmaceutical companies to, in effect, buy favorable drug reviews and weaken drug safety protections.

As Dr. Miller notes, the experiment with outside reviews was a success but the FDA lost interest under the Clinton administration.

After Republicans gained the majority in the Congress in 1994, they sought to streamline the FDA, particularly the process for the approval of new drugs. As the House of Representatives Commerce Committee staff member responsible for this effort, I drafted language for legislation that would have provided the FDA with the optional authority to approve new drugs based upon the recommendation of carefully regulated reviews conducted by outside experts. Using the same rigorous standards and requirements as FDA officials, expert reviewers authorized by the agency would have been able to conduct reviews to determine whether the data on new drugs met the criteria for safety and effectiveness—but only the FDA would have had the authority actually to approve a new drug, based on the recommendation of the extramural review. Almost half the members of Congress supported this concept.

Those opposed to extramural reviews argued that the use of private-sector experts raises potential problems of competence, integrity, and impartiality. Regrettably, this argument was generally accepted uncritically, in that no one presented actual evidence that private organizations performing tasks under government contracts and operating under appropriate safeguards are more susceptible to corruption than government officials. Critics of the proposal ignored or dismissed evidence that foreign governments with drug review organizations comparable to the United States widely, routinely, and effectively use nongovernmental individuals and organizations to conduct reviews of new drugs and medical devices. It is remarkable that those same critics have not objected when the FDA itself has sought outside expertise to help with certain routine reviews for medical devices or food products.

Contracting out various government functions is, of course, not novel. A large number of government functions—including many related to health and safety, environmental protection, and defense—are delegated to the private sector, and such arrangements are essential to the operation of the U.S. government. Indeed, many activities once performed by government are now delegated to private-sector contractors. It has been a long time since the government itself built navy ships and munitions. Federal agencies rely on a vast array of advisory committees composed of nongovernmental experts on various subjects. One prominent example is the reliance by the renowned National Institutes of Health on a large network of advisory committees consisting primarily of academic scientists, for advice on what extramural research should be funded.

In other areas the Clinton administration has proposed some privatization of government safety functions. For example, based on a recommendation of the National Performance Review for reinventing government, the administration has recommended the partial privatization of U.S. air traffic control and requested that the Department of Transportation develop a detailed action plan and statutory language for changes in the management of air traffic control that would make it more businesslike. However, the administration opposed the outside review of drug data favored by many in Congress, and the drug industry, possibly reluctant to antagonize those in power, was initially ambivalent and later actually averse to the concept. In the end, the opposition of the drug industry, the Clinton administration, and consumer activists derailed this FDA reform.

Although few Americans are aware of it, most of the process of drug development has always been conducted by the private sector. Industry, not the FDA, performs the discovery and clinical testing of new drugs under FDA rules. The results of a company's testing and other supporting information are submitted to the agency for review to determine whether the data support a conclusion that the drug meets the requirements for safety and effectiveness. This arrangement argues for the FDA's contracting out reviews: If integrity or competence of nongovernmental experts were an issue, the FDA should conduct its own research on new pharmaceuticals and not rely on industry studies. Opponents would argue, however, that it is exactly *because* pharmaceutical companies conduct the research that only government experts should review new drug applications as a check on any incompetence or misconduct. But this argument is weakened by the fact that nongovernmental reviewers are required to maintain standards of integrity and competence at least as high as those in government agencies, particularly since they are subject to legal liability for negligence. (The FDA's reviewers, however, are immune from such liability.) In the text, Dr. Miller discusses other factors that would protect the quality and integrity of nongovernmental reviewers and reviews.

The debate surrounding outside reviews may be as much about the FDA's desire to maintain its singular preeminence as about increasing the efficiency of the drug approval process. Yet the FDA has suffered from the types of problems associated with large monopolistic bureaucracies. For example, it failed to have systems in place to detect the corruption of some generic drug reviewers who in the 1980s accepted bribes to accelerate the approval of certain products and to delay others. It suffered again from high-profile dubious decisions such as the embargoing of Chilean grapes on the basis of exaggerated concerns about their safety, and the withdrawal from the market of silicone breast implants without clear scientific evidence of their risk. Dr. Miller notes other examples of dubious decision making and policymaking at the FDA.

Increasing the role of the private sector in the review of new drugs could well stimulate innovation in new drug development as well as make the new drug review process more efficient. Both would help to get more and better drugs to patients sooner. The successful Bush administration pilot study and the extensive experience of foreign governments have shown that nongovernmental reviewers have much to offer and that further efforts to take advantage of private resources should be pursued.

John J. Cohrssen
Executive Director, Public Health Policy Advisory Board
Formerly, Majority Counsel, House of Representatives
     Commerce Committee

Acknowledgments

The model described in this volume owes much to the landmark study of pharmaceutical regulation by the Washington, D.C.–based Progress & Freedom Foundation (PFF), "Advancing Medical Innovation: Health, Safety and the Role of Government in the 21st Century," which first described in 1996 a workable alternative to the government monopoly over the regulation of drug development. The current work expands the rationale and the context for such a proposal and describes them in greater detail.

I wish to thank all of my coauthors of the PFF study, particularly William M. Wardell, who for decades has studied and made significant contributions to the subject of regulatory reform, and Tom Lenard, who encouraged me to proceed with this sequel.

I thank Paula Duggan King, editrix extraordinaire, for both her patience and her editorial magic.

I am especially indebted to the Hoover Institution and its director, John Raisian, for funding my research and providing an extraordinary atmosphere in which to work.

Introduction

Medical technology has advanced at a stunning pace in the past half century, enabling drug and biotechnology companies to become major contributors of innovative life-saving and life-enhancing medicines. Scientific progress has yielded powerful tools such as rational drug design, combinatorial chemistry, gene-splicing, DNA-sequencing, and genomics that have wrought a creative revolution fueled by massive public- and private-sector investment. Since 1950 new vaccines have virtually eliminated measles, rubella, poliomyelitis, mumps, and diphtheria from the United States. Because of new antibiotics the child with bacterial meningitis can be snatched from death. Because of genetically engineered alfa interferon, the fifty-year-old with a rare type of leukemia can be successfully treated. Chemotherapy alone adds an average of nine years to the life of the testicular cancer patient.[1] To Americans with all kinds of potentially crippling health problems—from diabetes to multiple sclerosis to congestive heart failure—new drugs can give the gift of an all-but-normal daily life. The list of diseases and conditions that can be conquered or brought under control by new drug therapies is long and growing.

Furthermore, drugs can now improve both the span and the quality

1. Milton C. Weinstein and Janice C. Wright, "Gains in Life Expectancy from Medical Interventions," *Risk in Perspective* 6 (1998): 1–4.

of life in a surprisingly cost-effective way, a fact of crucial significance not only to the individual patient but to the nation as a whole: The responsible use of drug therapies lowers the total cost of health care. The National Bureau of Economic Research found, for example, that the overall cost of therapy for heart attacks and depression—both of which are commonly treated with drugs—actually declined by 1 percent each year from 1984 through 1991.[2] Similarly, the aggregate price of treating acute major depression fell by 25 percent from 1991 to 1995,[3] and studies of the impacts of a clot-dissolving drug in stroke patients[4] and a new drug for migraine headaches[5] show that these treatments too are highly cost-effective (see figures 1 and 2).

Advances in pharmaceuticals have produced a modern-day miracle. However, the miracle is not the subject of this book. My main concern is the obstacles to innovation that have arisen and incubated surreptitiously over time—the obstacles that can mitigate the miracle.

Inefficient and excessive regulation is one such obstacle. It has been with us for decades, and its consequences are now enormous. It threatens the leadership of the United States in drug discovery and development and the health and well-being of American citizens. It has pushed the costs of drug development to astronomical levels. Getting the average drug from the laboratory to a patient's bedside now requires twelve to fifteen years and costs more than $400 million,[6] with no gain in safety over countries whose regulation is more efficient and less costly. These costs have caused a significant ripple effect in the American

2. David Cutler, Mark McClellan, and Joseph Newhouse, *The Costs and Benefits of Intensive Treatment for Cardiovascular Disease* (Washington, D.C.: American Enterprise Institute for Public Policy Research/Brookings Institution, December 1997).

3. Richard G. Frank, Ernst Berndt, and Susan H. Busch, *Price Indexes for the Treatment of Depression* (Washington D.C.: American Enterprise Institute for Public Policy Research/Brookings Institution, December 1997).

4. Susan C. Fagan et al., "Cost-effectiveness of Tissue Plasminogen Activator for Acute Ischemic Stroke," *Neurology* 50 (1998): 883–89.

5. Randall F. Legg et al., "Cost Benefit of Sumatriptan to an Employer," *Journal of Occupational and Environmental Medicine* 39 (1997): 652–57.

6. Office of Technology Assessment, U.S. Congress, *Pharmaceutical R&D: Costs, Risks and Rewards* (Washington, D.C.: U.S. Government Printing Office, 1993).

Millions of Dollars per 1,000 Patients

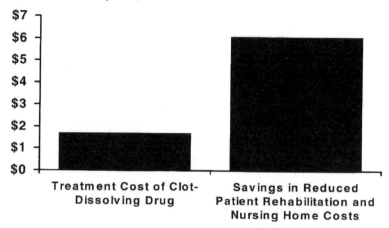

Figure 1.   Costs and Saving of Using Clot-Dissolving Drug.
Source: Pharmaceutical Research and Manufacturers of America, *1999 Industry Profile* (Washington, D.C.: PhRMA, 1999). (Original data from Susan C. Fagan et al., "Cost-effectiveness of Tissue Plasminogen Activator for Acute Ischemic Stroke," *Neurology* 50 [1998]: 883–90.)

pharmaceutical industry: corporate consolidations, lessened competition, higher retail prices, and an increasing tendency to develop only sure things—that is, lower-risk research projects that are intended for large patient populations and highly likely to pass regulatory scrutiny—even if they advance medical science only minimally. It is significant that during the 1960s cancer patients in the United States had more therapeutic agents available to them than did patients in Great Britain, Germany, France, or Japan; now they have fewer.

Defenders of the present regulatory system in this country argue that lower efficiency is the price of safety. But this doesn't have to be true. High standards of safety and greater efficiency are both achievable if we are willing to reform fundamentally the way drugs are regulated. If we can end regulatory excesses, introduce competition into regulatory oversight, and redirect government involvement to those few activities where a central, monopolistic role is essential, more patients will benefit from a greater number of drugs made available to them in a timelier way.

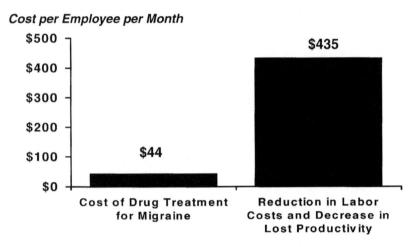

Figure 2.   Labor Costs and Levels of Productivity Using Drug Treatment for Migraine. *Source:* Pharmaceutical Research and Manufacturers of America, *1999 Industry Profile* (Washington, D.C.: PhRMA, 1999). (Original data from Randall F. Legg et al., "Cost Benefit of Sumatriptan to an Employer," *Journal of Occupational and Environmental Medicine* 39 [1997]: 652–57.)

Since the present system for the regulation of drugs in the United States was established in 1962 under the aegis of the Food and Drug Administration (FDA), this agency has inexorably increased its responsibilities and intrusiveness, along with its regulatory demands on drug manufacturers. The costs and delays of research and development have increased concomitantly, leading to a broad consensus among physicians, public policy analysts, and others familiar with drug regulation that the FDA imposes far more expansive and stringent regulation on pharmaceuticals than is warranted. Numerous independent analyses, including comparisons of the FDA with drug regulators abroad, have produced recommendations for improvements that would reduce the time, cost, complexity, and unpredictability of the research and development process.[7] None of these recommendations has come close to

7. Sheila R. Shulman, Peg Hewitt, and Michael Manocchia, "Studies and Inquiries into the FDA Regulatory Process: An Historical Review," *Drug Information Journal* 29, no. 2 (April–June 1995): 385–413.

fundamental reform, however; most of them have merely tinkered at the margins of the existing system. Even the much-touted Food and Drug Modernization Act of 1997 (FDAMA) did little more than codify what was already in place.

It is in the public interest to spur innovation in the discovery, development, and marketing of new diagnostics and therapies, to stimulate vigorous competition among manufacturers, and to have an efficient system of oversight. Why, then, should we tolerate a monopoly over drug regulation when we know that monopolies, whether in the public or private sector, encourage complacency, inefficiency, and ever-expanding bureaucracies?

The current system of drug regulation is, literally, overkill and works against the public interest. But if this is so, skeptics will ask, why is there no sense of urgency, no public outrage? Why is there no lobbying effort for regulatory reform from any prominent quarter or interest group? The reasons for this are complex. Would-be reformers are often accused of being beholden to drug manufacturers and of plotting deregulation, which is seen as capitulation to big business. Paradoxically, however, the biggest pharmaceutical companies are themselves *not* lobbying for reform. Why not?

First, American drug companies continue to be profitable. For them the huge expenses pertaining to regulation are simply part of the costs of doing business—and their own massive regulatory-affairs bureaucracies have become, in effect, special interests that feel they are not best served by less regulation. Excessive, rigid regulation is advantageous to larger companies because it discriminates against smaller ones, the principal innovators in drug development. The smaller companies feel the burden of excessive regulation more acutely and are more eager for regulatory change; but even for them regulatory reform is, at most, a long-term strategic goal, and they are more concerned with day-to-day crises. Moreover, individually they are ill equipped—and probably ill advised—to tackle the agency that holds the key to their futures. Trade associations are better able to be aggressive, to pressure regulators for reforms or other concessions (inasmuch as, unlike individual companies, they are largely immune from retribution), but the two major trade associations representing American pharmaceutical companies—the Pharmaceutical Research and Manufacturers of America and the Biotechnology Industry Organization—are dominated by large companies and have not been aggressive about regulatory reform. Second, despite all the obstacles, entrepreneurial ingenuity superimposed on technological innovation continues to spawn new companies. A wave of new start-ups is launched with each new technology or scientific breakthrough. This happened with the advent of gene-splicing and hybridoma technology in the 1970s and more recently with antisense technology, human gene therapy, and the availability of data from sequencing of the human genome. Even Everest-like regulatory barriers cannot exterminate the drive to create, compete, and succeed in this field.

For different equally complex reasons, the American public is just as passive as the drug companies about regulatory reform. Although it is literally dying for it, the aging American population is not clamoring for a more streamlined, responsive system that will offer it more new drugs at lower cost. For one thing, few Americans now pay the full costs of pharmaceuticals out of pocket. A significant fraction of prescription drug costs are absorbed by some kind of third-party payer, usually a managed-care organization or insurance company. Therefore, notwithstanding the occasional TV exposé that shows a retiree paying as much for drugs as for rent, individuals who need expensive new drugs seldom feel acutely the impact of inflated prices at the pharmacy.

Second, as far as most of the public is concerned, the nuances of drug development and its regulation are quite arcane and obscure. For example, many people assume that the FDA actually carries out the testing of pharmaceuticals, but it does not; the agency only evaluates data generated and submitted by industry. And the media has done little to educate them. Too often, the media evince interest in regulatory affairs only during a crisis—or what they can portray as one. (Their motto: If it bleeds it leads.) Even consumers who have a rudimentary understanding of who does what to whom in the process of drug development and its regulation tend to be fearful about new products. Americans have been conditioned to seek technological innovation that is completely risk free and to seek someone to blame when it is not. They are misled by drug detractors and biotechnology bashers who regularly raise false alarms and demand that regulators ban, withdraw, limit, and restrict all manner of safe and useful products.

These factors combine to confuse consumers and make them hesitant even to endorse, let alone demand, significant regulatory reform. Not realizing that there is a point of vanishing returns, which we have long since passed, they tend to believe that more regulation must be synonymous with more protection, that more government scrutiny will lower our risks. In addition, since there is a lack of sound, objective, easily accessible information about the potential harmfulness of the regulatory status quo, they exhibit "rational apathy," which simply means that in the absence of any obvious and proximate threat to their well-being it is reasonable for them to remain unconcerned.

Another phenomenon comes into play here: Major societal changes seldom occur except at times of crisis, when, it has been said, ideas have consequences. As Nobelist Milton Friedman observed, in a kind of economist's formulation of the physical property of inertia, "once a tide in opinion or in affairs is strongly set, it tends to overwhelm countercurrents and to keep going for a long time in the same direction. The tides are capable of ignoring geography, political labels, and other hindrances to their continuance."[8] Yet, Friedman continues, the very success of these tides "tends to create conditions that may ultimately reverse them."

No matter how profound the economic and public health costs of overregulation, no matter how potent and lucid the arguments for

---

8. Milton Friedman and Rose D. Friedman, "The Tide in the Affairs of Men," in Annelise Anderson and Dennis L. Bark, eds., *Thinking About America: The United States in the 1990s* (Stanford: Hoover Institution Press, 1988), p. 467.

regulatory reform, unless the public demands it—or at least begins to understand its potential benefits—fundamental changes are unlikely to occur.

The purpose of this volume is to stimulate, in two ways, a counter-current to the prevailing flood tide of monopolistic overregulation of drug development—first, by presenting evidence that the existing system is flawed and needs fundamental reform (part 1) and, second, by describing a coherent, comprehensive proposal for the form it should take (part 2). The purpose is not to be alarmist but to describe existing conditions—and possibilities for change—in a way that might eventually turn the tide.

PART I

THE NEED FOR FUNDAMENTAL FOOD AND DRUG ADMINISTRATION REFORM

1

The Birth and Growth of
Premarket Regulation

The federal government's role in regulating consumer products today is so pervasive that most Americans probably assume it is one of Washington's basic, essential jobs—like building highways and collecting taxes. Every consumer product sold is subject to at least one, and in many instances several, federal regulatory statutes, plus a bewildering array of implementing regulations, guidelines, and policies. But these regulations are relatively recent phenomena; before the twentieth century, in fact, there was no direct federal regulation of consumer products in the United States.

The Biologics Act of 1902 ushered in the Regulatory Century, and, as is often the case with regulatory legislation, it was written in a crisis atmosphere. In 1901, a contaminated smallpox vaccine caused an outbreak of tetanus in Camden, New Jersey, and a single lot of tetanus-contaminated diphtheria antitoxin resulted in the death of several children in St. Louis. Ensuing petitions triggered historic legislation. The 1902 statute required that the federal government grant *pre*market approval of two complementary license applications for every biological drug (blood and blood products, vaccines, derivatives of natural sub-

This section was adapted from the foreword by Peter Barton Hutt to Henry I. Miller, *Policy Controversy in Biotechnology: An Insider's View* (Austin, Tex.: R. G. Landes, 1997), with permission of the publisher.

stances for treating allergies, and extracts of living cells). One application was a product license application (certifying the product itself); the other was an establishment license application (validating the production process and facility). Never before had any European or American government required explicit government licensing or approval of a category of consumer products before marketing.[1] Earlier lawmaking in Europe, the American colonies, and the United States had made the sale of adulterated or misbranded products illegal but had provided governmental authorities only with the power to police the marketplace; that is, regulators could review already marketed products and bring legal action against any product found to violate the statutory requirements. With the 1902 act, government was given the unprecedented administrative authority to prevent the marketing of a consumer product. It could bar the product from ever reaching the marketplace simply by turning down a marketing application or by taking no action at all on the matter. The same premarket authority was later enacted into law for animal biological drugs, in the Virus, Serum, and Toxin Act of 1913.

Congress did not grant this power casually; in fact, the premarket approval requirements of the Biologics Act of 1902 stood alone for more than fifty years. When Congress enacted the Federal Food and Drugs Act of 1906 to regulate the rest of the drug supply (that is, nonbiological drugs) in the United States, it did not authorize any form of premarket testing or approval or even the development of administrative regulatory standards. The Federal Meat Inspection Act of 1906 and the Insecticide Act of 1910 similarly relied entirely on traditional police powers and imposed no regulatory requirements before marketing.

As first drafted, even the Federal Food, Drug and Cosmetic Act of 1938—the principal enabling statue of today's FDA—included only policing authority. Before it became law, however, a hastily marketed drug containing an untested solvent (diethylene glycol, a potent poison) killed more than a hundred people within a few days. In response to

---

1. Peter Barton Hutt, foreword, in Henry I. Miller, *Policy Controversy in Biotechnology: An Insider's View* (Austin, Tex.: R. G. Landes, 1997).

this tragedy, Congress included in the 1938 act a new provision to require sponsors (companies) to submit a New Drug Application (NDA) to the FDA before introducing a new drug into interstate commerce. The NDA described the proposed uses of the drug and the tests that demonstrated safety at the recommended dose. Under the 1938 act, if a company submitted an NDA for a product and the FDA took no action within sixty days, the application was, in effect, approved and the drug could be marketed lawfully. In other words, Congress stopped short of requiring that new drugs obtain an *affirmative* premarket approval; the default position was permission for the drug sponsor to market the product. Moreover, only the safety, not the effectiveness, of the drug was considered to be within the FDA's purview; effectiveness was left for the marketplace to determine.

A decade later, following World War II, Congress replaced the Insecticide Act of 1910 with the Federal Insecticide, Fungicide, and Rodenticide Act (FIFRA) of 1947. For the first time, every pesticide was required to be registered before it could be marketed lawfully. The 1947 act contained no authority, however, for the United States Department of Agriculture (USDA), which regulated pesticides at that time, to deny registration based on an administrative determination that a product was adulterated or mislabeled.

The combined impact of these various federal regulatory statutes on commerce in legitimate products was negligible, and there were, in fact, public health benefits. The policing, or surveillance, of the marketplace—that is, *postmarket* regulation—by the FDA and USDA under these regulatory statutes was extremely successful in weeding out adulterated and misbranded products. By taking strong regulatory action, these two agencies removed thousands of unsafe and ineffective products from the market, thus benefiting both consumers and the legitimate industry. At the same time neither the industry's ability to develop and market new products nor individual choice were compromised: Because their scope was narrow, the premarket approval requirements for human and animal biological products had little negative impact, and free choice in the marketplace was actually enhanced by the requirement for accurate labeling of regulated products.

Beginning in the 1950s, however, the regulatory landscape changed dramatically. Congress required premarket approval of a large number of consumer products by enacting the following series of statutes:

- Miller Pesticide Amendments of 1954, requiring premarket approval of pesticide residues in or on food

- Food Additives Amendment of 1958, requiring premarket approval of food additives

- Color Additive Amendments of 1960, requiring premarket approval of color additives

- Drug Amendments of 1962, which introduced premarket affirmative approval and required that marketed drugs be found by the FDA to be both safe *and effective*

- Animal Drug Amendments of 1968, requiring premarket approval of new animal drugs and feed additives

- Federal Environmental Pesticide Control Act of 1972, requiring premarket approval of pesticides

- Medical Device Amendments of 1976, requiring premarket notification for all medical devices and premarket approval for Class III medical devices

- Toxic Substances Control Act of 1976, requiring premarket notification for chemical substances

- Infant Formula Act of 1980, requiring premarket notification for infant formulas

- Nutrition Labeling and Education Act of 1990, requiring premarket approval of nutrient descriptors and disease prevention claims for food

The pivotal event in U.S. drug regulation was passage of the 1962 amendments to the Food, Drug and Cosmetic Act of 1938. Whereas under the 1938 statute a product could be marketed unless the FDA actually denied approval of the NDA, after 1962 an affirmative approval from the agency was required; in other words, disapproval was the default position. The 1962 statute also imposed other significant constraints and requirements on drug sponsors: For the first time, all human testing of new drugs, all drug advertising, and all labeling had to be reviewed and precleared by the FDA, and the FDA promulgated Good Manufacturing Practices regulations.[2] The Food, Drug and Cosmetic Act, as amended, fundamentally altered the nature of American drug research, development, and production. Judgments about what was desirable and undesirable could no longer be made primarily by manufacturers, physicians, and patients via the marketplace but were entrusted to a regulatory monopoly administered by a central governmental authority.

The enormous economic impact on pharmaceuticals was seen almost immediately after the 1962 law was enacted. The drug industry's research output declined rapidly, as measured by the introduction of Investigational New Drug (IND) Applications to the FDA to begin clinical testing for new chemical entities (NCEs). There was an immediate decline of more than 50 percent in the early 1960s; for about a decade thereafter the output was fairly constant, but in the mid-1970s it fell again by another 50 percent. The submission rate recovered somewhat in the early 1980s but declined again from the mid-1980s to the mid-1990s.[3] (Since about 1990, the shortfall in INDs for NCEs has been compensated for by an increase in the introduction of INDs for biotechnology products, which are predominantly biological drugs and are, for historical reasons, not counted as NCEs.) Another effect of the

2. Henry G. Grabowski and John M. Vernon, *The Regulation of Pharmaceuticals* (Washington, D.C.: American Enterprise Institute for Public Policy Research, 1983), pp. 2–4.

3. Joseph DiMasi, M. A. Seibring, and Louis Lasagna, "New Drug Development in the United States, 1963 to 1992," *Clinical Pharmacology and Therapeutics* 55 (1994): 609–22.

increasingly onerous and unpredictable regulatory requirements in the United States is that many American companies have chosen to test and market their products abroad. Reflecting this migration are the disproportionate increases abroad in numbers of employees of American research-based pharmaceutical companies, as compared to U.S.-based employees. From December 1995 to June 1998, for example, foreign employment by these companies grew by 17.2 percent, while domestic employment increased 4.8 percent.[4] (The fact that there was an actual *decrease* of 10.2 percent in the numbers of domestic scientific, professional, and technical staff in American research-based companies from 1995 through 1997, the last time period for which statistics are available, argues that this is unlikely to be a reflection of shifts in marketing, sales, and administrative personnel.[5] In other words, there has been a real redistribution of scientific and technical resources.)

The other legislative actions enumerated above did to most other commercial sectors what the 1962 amendments did to drug regulation. Taken collectively, this legislation has resulted in a revolution in product regulation. Since the 1950s federal responsibility has grown from simple policing after the product launch to virtually universal premarket regulation.

Possessing a monopoly on product review and approval, the federal government has in most sectors become the sole gatekeeper to the marketplace; regulators at a veritable alphabet soup of agencies now have the final authority to determine whether and when a product will reach consumers. For a product subject to premarket approval, no manufacturer has the legal right to distribute the product and no member of the public has the right to obtain it, unless and until the relevant federal agency authorizes marketing. Statute by statute, regulation by regulation, and decision by decision, massive bureaucracies have arisen to rein in industry and control product flow. What many fail to realize

4. Pharmaceutical Research and Manufacturers of America, *Pharmaceutical Industry 1999* (Washington, D.C.: Pharmaceutical Research and Manufacturers of America), pp. 113–15.
    5. Ibid.

is that a regulatory statute, even if it is not amended, is not static. When the statute is first enacted, its implementation is generally narrow and limited to the specific requirements of the law, and its impact, therefore, is often modest. As time goes on, however, each successive generation of administrators tends to redefine the scope of jurisdiction and add new requirements. Seldom does the scope narrow; almost never do requirements disappear. Regulation begins to take on a life of its own. And as regulators interpret statutes ever more broadly and comprehensively, they become, in effect, a special interest group with a vested interest in expanded responsibilities, budgets, and empires. In the absence of effective, conscientious congressional oversight, what develops is an increasingly burdensome and inefficient regulatory system. Nowhere can this be seen more clearly than in the evolution of premarket licensing mechanisms for drugs.

The current system of oversight of pharmaceutical development includes no mechanism for public accountability. This means, for example, that citizens who could benefit from certain pharmaceutical products have no right to participate in the process and no access to judicial review of whatever action is taken by the federal government. Even the applicant (company) is precluded from access to the courts until final action is taken on a product application. And neither the public nor the media readily learns about potentially life-saving drugs and devices that have been delayed by regulators' timidity or foot-dragging. Thus, premarket approval severely limits individual freedom of choice. Personal autonomy is subjugated to government controls. Citizens are precluded from obtaining products they wish to purchase and have no recourse other than to await government approval. American citizens have been forced to travel abroad to obtain drugs and treatments not available in the United States because of our slower and more stringent regulatory system, and they have even been prohibited from bringing these drugs back into this country for their own use.

When combined with other economic consequences of regulation, these constraints on patient access create an invisible crisis. The greater the investment required to bring products to market, the less competition there is to make them, so fewer products are pursued and the price to consumers for the products that are ultimately approved steadily increases. Particularly for small businesses, the investment required to obtain premarket approval of products such as drugs and pesticides can be prohibitive. Although there have been other challenges as well to entrepreneurship and corporate innovation in the pharmaceutical industry—some of which are discussed in subsequent chapters—increased regulatory requirements, the FDA's risk-averse culture, and the absence of effective congressional oversight of drug regulators have been major impediments.

2

Factors Affecting
Drug Development

Regulatory Creep at the FDA

The FDA is arguably the most omnipresent regulatory agency in the United States. It has responsibility for more than a trillion dollars worth of consumer products annually, ranging from condoms and X-ray machines to drugs, vaccines, pregnancy home-testing kits, and artificial sweeteners. In its role as the nation's regulator of drugs, the agency is the gatekeeper between the developer and the marketplace.

The FDA's enabling statutes—the Federal Food, Drug and Cosmetic Act and the Public Health Service Act (which mandates regulation of biological drugs)—are not highly prescriptive or detailed. They permit government regulators great latitude to apply scientific knowledge and common sense to oversight. However, this latitude has also freed regulators to decide how much power and discretion they should exercise. Not surprisingly, their tendency has been consistently toward ever greater power and discretion.

The FDA evaluates and approves drugs. It does not discover or test them. That is done by a sponsor, usually a private pharmaceutical company. This point can not be overemphasized: It is not the FDA that is bringing life-saving new therapies to American consumers but private companies and research institutions. The process of research and development is difficult in the best of circumstances—and not always

financially rewarding—so the relationship between sponsor and overseer is critical in ensuring that consumers reap all the health benefits
possible in a timely and safe manner. Development of a new drug begins
with *preclinical* investigations: in vitro screening for a desired chemical
or biological activity or trait, followed by screening in laboratory animals
to determine therapeutic activity and possible toxicity. These preclinical
investigations generate preliminary knowledge about the pharmacological and toxicological properties of the agent. If they yield promising
results, they are followed by *clinical testing* in humans over a period of
years. Two obligatory applications to the FDA are made as part of the
process of drug development. Before embarking on the first phase of
clinical testing, the sponsor must submit an application called an Investigational New Drug, or IND, filing. The agency then monitors the
testing through periodic reports, inspections and audits. When clinical
testing has progressed to a point where the drug sponsor is satisfied that
the drug is ready for consumers and meets the regulatory standards of
safety and effectiveness for a specific use, it submits the second man-
datory application, the New Drug Application, or NDA, seeking approval to market the drug.

Rather than guiding and facilitating this process the FDA often ob-
structs it. The agency constantly promulgates new requirements—or
seemingly arbitrary interpretations of old requirements—with apparent
disregard for the costs to patients and regulated industry. One measure
of these increasingly expansive and rigorous requirements is the growing
number of clinical trials during drug development. Since 1980, the
average number of clinical trials conducted to support an NDA has
more than doubled, from thirty to almost seventy (see figure 3).[1] Likewise, the average number of patients required to support an NDA has
increased almost threefold, from 1,576 in the late 1970s to 4,237 in the
mid-1990s (see figure 4),[2] and the number of medical procedures during

1. Carl C. Peck, "Drug Development: Improving the Process," *Food & Drug Law
Journal* (1997): 163–67.
2. Pharmaceutical Research and Manufacturers of America, *1999 Industry Profile*
(Washington, D.C.: PhRMA, 1999), p. 32.

Number of Trials

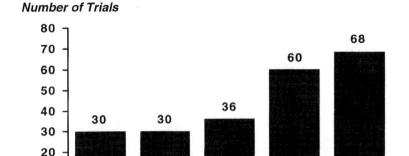

Figure 3. Average Number of Clinical Trials per New Drug Application. *Source:* Pharmaceutical Research and Manufacturers of America, *1999 Industry Profile* (Washington, D.C.: PhRMA, 1999). (Original data from Boston Consulting Group, "The Contribution of Pharmaceutical Companies: What's at Stake for America," Boston, September 1993; and Carl C. Peck, "Drug Development: Improving the Process,"*Food & Drug Law Journal* [1997]: 163–67.)

clinical trials rose 61 percent from 1992 to 1997.[3] These costs add up. DiMasi, Hansen, and Grabowski estimated in 1991 that the cost of bringing the average drug to market was $231 million (in 1987 dollars).[4] Using the same data but a higher discount rate, the congressional Office of Technology Assessment in 1993 estimated the cost as $359 million (in 1990 dollars).[5] Adjusted for inflation, these figures (in 1998 dollars) would now be $313 million and $432 million, respectively, to develop a single drug—the highest price tag in the world. The figure is un-questionably much higher now: Chasing these skyrocketing costs, just between 1994 and 1996 U.S. research-based drug companies'

3. Ibid., p. 33.
4. Joseph A. DiMasi et al., "Cost of Innovation in the Pharmaceutical Industry," *Journal of Health Economics* 10 (1991): 108–42.
5. Office of Technology Assessment, U.S. Congress, *Pharmaceutical R&D: Costs, Risks and Rewards* (Washington, D.C.: U.S. Government Printing Office, 1993).

Number of Patients

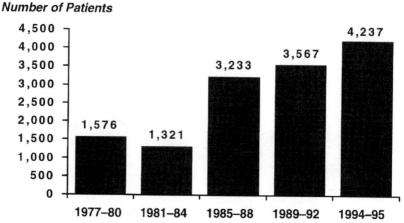

Figure 4. Average Number of Patients per New Drug Application.
Source: Pharmaceutical Research and Manufacturers of America, *1999 Industry Profile* (Washington, D.C.: PhRMA, 1999). (Original data from Boston Consulting Group, "The Contribution of Pharmaceutical Companies: What's at Stake for America," Boston, September 1993; and Carl C. Peck, "Drug Development: Improving the Process," *Food & Drug Law Journal* [1997]: 163–67.)

expenditures on clinical trials increased 32 percent, and their expenditures on regulatory affairs to support research and development increased 29 percent.[6] A 1994 study at Duke University revealed a sobering corollary to these findings: During the period 1980–1984, only three out of every ten drug products produced revenues that covered their development costs (see figure 5).[7] The researchers also found that the 20 percent of products with the highest revenues generated 70 percent of the returns. In other words, because of the high cost and high risk of drug research, companies must rely on a limited number of highly successful products to finance their continuing research and development.

6. Pharmaceutical Research and Manufacturers Association, *New Drug Approvals* (Washington, D.C.: Pharmaceutical Research and Manufacturers Association, January 1998), pp. 18–21.
7. Henry G. Grabowski and John M. Vernon, "Returns to R&D on New Drug Introductions in the 1980s," *Journal of Health Economics* 13 (1994): 383–406.

Millions of 1990 Dollars

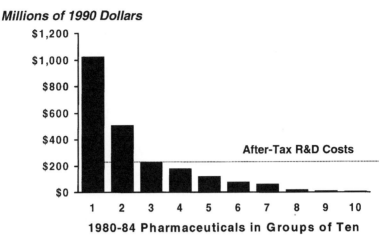

Figure 5. Drugs' Revenues Compared to Research and Development (R&D) Costs. *Source:* Pharmaceutical Research and Manufacturers of America, *1999 Industry Profile* (Washington, D.C.: PhRMA, 1999). (Original data from Henry G. Grabowski and John M. Vernon, *The Regulation of Pharmaceuticals* [Washington, D.C.: American Enterprise Institute for Public Policy Research, 1983], pp. 2–4.)

The converse should also be true: More modest regulatory costs would reduce the pressure on the research-based drug companies to bring forth blockbusters, making it possible for them to afford to develop more products whose revenues will be modest. In other words, if costs were lower, manufacturers would pursue a greater number of products.

Why Is Drug Development So Expensive and Slow?

The FDA constantly raises the bar for the initiation and progress of clinical testing of new drugs. For example, in just the past few years FDA officials have arbitrarily and unexpectedly directed clinical investigators to begin trials at inappropriately low dosages; limited approval of phase I studies only to single-dose, instead of dose-ranging, studies; demanded unnecessary, invasive procedures on patients; and even required that foreign trials be completed and the results submitted before the U.S. trials could begin. The 1999 death of a patient in a gene-therapy trial at the University of Pennsylvania offers an example of overreaction by the FDA and its consequences. Although the cause of the multiorgan failure in the teenage patient had not been determined, the FDA tightened manufacturing standards for academic investigators, inaccurately but publicly accused the clinical investigators of various kinds of mistakes and misconduct, shut down all the university's gene-therapy trials, and even halted trials being performed by a drug company using a similar preparation.[8] The FDA's precipitous actions following a single unexplained death during a trial cast a pall on gene-therapy research throughout the country and discouraged commercial support for the field.

This constant raising of the bar has made the drug development process in the United States the lengthiest in the world, and it grows longer all the time. According to the Tufts University Center for the Study of Drug Development, since the 1960s the total time required for drug development—from synthesis or discovery in the laboratory to the patient's bedside—has almost doubled, from 8.1 years to 15.2 years.[9] Clinical testing, the portion of the development process most intensely scrutinized by the FDA, averages eight years in the United States, about a third longer than in Europe.

Another source of frustration to drug sponsors is that, as the time required for drug development has lengthened, the average effective patent life—that is, the time span between NDA approval and expiration of the main patent—has declined correspondingly. Despite twenty-year U.S. patent terms, the average period of the useful (post-FDA approval) patent life of new drugs introduced in the 1990s was only eleven to twelve years.[10] Under current law, some of the time lost to FDA review may be recaptured by the holder of the patent but only up to a total of

8. Henry I. Miller, "Gene Therapy's Trials and Tribulations," *The Scientist*, February 7, 2000, p. 16.

9. The Tufts University Center for the Study of Drug Development, *1996–97 Annual Report* (Boston: Tufts University, 1997).

10. Pharmaceutical Research and Manufacturers of America, *1999 Industry Profile* (Washington, D.C.: PhRMA, 1999), pp 83–87.

fourteen years, and the legislation that permitted this adjustment exacted substantial, costly concessions from the research-based drug industry, including earlier approval of generic drugs. This situation compares unfavorably to other industries, where companies receive an average of eighteen and a half years of effective patent protection.

In other words, overregulation and truncated patent life are double disincentives for anyone considering drug development.

Does Slowness = Safety?

The FDA's regulatory regimes are sometimes referred to as the world's gold standard, meaning that the agency's standards are the most difficult to meet and implying that FDA-approved products are, therefore, the safest. Defenders of this myth of the supremacy of the FDA—and the status quo—argue that a slow and expensive regulatory regime is the price that must be paid for a high degree of safety. However, that argument does not justify a system that wholly ignores the opportunity costs of inefficient, unnecessarily burdensome regulation. These are real costs. Public health is harmed when potentially beneficial products are delayed, abandoned, or never tested at all.

Consider the delay in the marketing of the currently used, second generation of hepatitis B vaccines. The first hepatitis B vaccine came from an unlikely and precarious source—the pooled plasma of patients with chronic active hepatitis, which is likely to contain live, infectious hepatitis B virus and other viruses. Each batch was purified and treated to inactivate any infectious agents that might be present, and the product was judged safe and effective and licensed by the FDA in 1982. Nevertheless, neither patients nor physicians were enthusiastic about the product, and it was not widely used.

When a few years later Merck & Company developed a candidate for a second-generation vaccine that was genetically engineered—by introducing a single gene from the hepatitis B virus into baker's yeast— there was great anticipation and excitement: Because no live virus or human fluids were used in the manufacturing process, the probability of contamination with infectious viruses was virtually zero. Therefore, safety was only a secondary issue, and the pivotal policy question for the FDA was what should be the criteria for evaluating the efficacy of this new product. The most conservative of the several options was extensive clinical trials in susceptible patient groups in order to demonstrate conclusively that the vaccine would actually prevent hepatitis. This option was also the most expensive. Such trials could only be conducted in Asia, where a sufficiently high natural incidence of the disease means that one can readily see a statistically significant effect in clinical trials, but such trials take a long time. An alternative to requiring prevention of hepatitis as the clinical end point was the use of surrogate end points short of actual disease prevention. For example, it was known from use of the first-generation vaccine that certain levels and kinds of antibodies correlate with immunity. The adoption of these surrogate end points would have meant measuring the ability of the vaccine to elicit the appropriate levels and kinds of antibodies. Still another option would have charted a middle course (which, as an FDA medical officer at the time, I favored). This option relied primarily on antibody studies but included a small, confirmatory clinical trial (which could have been completed after the licensing of the vaccine) to demonstrate actual prevention of disease. Because there were no serious safety concerns about the genetically engineered vaccine, this middle course seemed prudent: After the demonstration of an appropriate immune response and preliminary clinical evidence that the vaccine conferred resistance to hepatitis, it would be made available to the public while more comprehensive studies were in progress.

Characteristically, in the end the FDA adopted the most risk-averse course: massive clinical trials in Asia, involving thousands of patients and the expenditure of tens of millions of dollars. This decision meant a delay of several years in getting the product to market. During that period of delay, while only the inferior, seldom-used, first-generation vaccine was available, more than ten thousand Americans unnecessarily contracted hepatitis B. Some of these patients died from complications of the disease, such as cirrhosis and hepatic carcinoma. Recombivax®, the second-generation vaccine, reduced the incidence of hepatitis B by 65 percent during the decade following its approval in 1986 (see figure 6).

Another myth about the supposedly inevitable link between slowness and safety in drug regulation holds that the more stringent regulatory policies of the United States afford greater protection from drug-related adverse effects, such as toxicities that are unknown at the time of marketing approval but discovered after extensive use of the drug. Although data are not yet available for comparisons of safety discontinuations (removals from the market) between the FDA and its European equivalent, the European Agency for the Evaluation of Medicinal Products (EMEA), there have been comparisons between the United States and the United Kingdom (whose approach is similar to the EMEA). Bakke et al. found that while the number of safety discontinuations in the United Kingdom was larger than in the United States, the overall number of drugs approved in the United Kingdom was also larger.[11] As a result, the numbers of safety discontinuations as a percentage of total new drug introductions in each country were similar—approximately 4 percent in the United Kingdom versus about 3 percent in the United States. In other words, the probability that a marketed drug will be removed from the market is not appreciably different in the United Kingdom and United States.

New Factors (Should) Make the FDA Less Important

Although any system of drug oversight should preserve a high degree of assurance of product safety and efficacy, such assurance comes increasingly not only through federal regulation but from the evolving interplay among industry, government, academia, and medical practice. Since

---

11. Olav M. Bakke, William M. Wardell, and Louis Lasagna, "Drug Discontinuations in the United Kingdom and the United States, 1964 to 1983: Issues of Safety," *Clinical Pharmacology and Therapeutics* 35 (1984): 559–67.

Cases per 100,000 Population

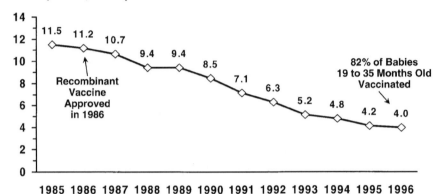

Figure 6. Effect of Vaccine on Incidence of Hepatitis B.
Source: Pharmaceutical Research and Manufacturers of America, *1999 Industry Profile* (Washington, D.C.: PhRMA, 1999). (Original data from Centers for Disease Control and Prevention, U.S. Department of Health and Human Services, 1998.)

the current framework for the regulation of new drug development was put in place four decades ago, basic and clinical research techniques have advanced, the media have become both more aggressive and more attuned to health issues—if not to drug regulation specifically—and public sophistication and awareness about general health concerns have grown. In addition, pharmaceutical marketing, tort case law, and the system for cost reimbursement for medical treatments have all changed dramatically. These factors have changed the manufacturer-physician-patient relationship and added layers of analysis and control to the FDA evaluation and approval process.

There are many more professional, full-time, career clinical research-ers now than in the 1960s, and also more proficient, for-profit clinical research organizations that design and perform clinical studies for drug sponsors. In addition, there has been a proliferation of institutional safeguards to patients, such as corporate mechanisms for carrying out and overseeing clinical trials and conducting postmarketing drug sur-veillance, and the (government-mandated) establishment of institutional review boards (IRBs) in clinical research institutions. The reporting of adverse events (side effects) has been improved—although arguably this pharmacovigilance needs further strengthening—and a new science, pharmacoepidemiology, systematically examines adverse events in exposed populations. But the most profound changes have resulted from the evolution of various nongovernmental entities into de facto drug-vetting, standard-setting organizations. The newest and most potent of these are managed-care organizations, which exercise their influence through large-scale purchasing, monitoring, formularies, and drug utilization review. The ability of physicians practicing within such organizations to prescribe is increasingly affected and constrained by computerized systems (governors) that perform overall integration of the medical record for case management. A physician can be prevented from prescribing medication if, for example, according to computerized monitoring of his decisions, the drug is inconsistent with a patient's listed diagnosis; excessive in dose, frequency, or length of administration; or likely to interact dangerously with another medication the patient is taking. In addition, drugs can be omitted or removed from formularies when cheaper alternatives become available or when they are deemed to be nonessential because they treat conditions like baldness or wrinkles or only aid the cessation of smoking. In a sense the HMO has become a second gatekeeper between the manufacturer and the patient.

A manufacturer used to be able to encourage individual physicians directly to prescribe a new drug, via advertising in journals and through the distribution of samples and other perquisites. Now a product typically must undergo pharmacoeconomics analysis and survive the vetting of a panel of experts who comprise a managed-care organization's formulary committee. A reflection of these new criteria, which exceed the FDA's already stringent requirements for safety and efficacy, is the growth of pharmacoeconomics departments in drug companies and their involvement in decision making related to research and development. These departments have become involved in evaluating licensing opportunities, selecting compounds for clinical development, and deciding on the termination of research on individual products.[12] To succeed in today's marketplace, manufacturers' products and claims, and the evidence supporting them, must meet a broad spectrum of standards. And at the same time, a system of judicial restraint and punishment of drug manufacturers has developed that further constrains drug discovery and development.

These various extragovernmental mechanisms and developments work in concert to protect the integrity of the clinical trials and, after approval, to assure product safety, efficacy, and effective postmarketing surveillance. Arguably, the operation of these factors diminishes the relative importance of the FDA as the protector of the patient. Taking the argument further, one might even postulate that in the complete absence of a governmental drug-regulating agency, market forces would spur the creation of whatever mechanisms would be required to assess and ensure pharmaceuticals' safety and efficacy. This is, after all, what *Consumer Reports*, *Consumers' Research*, J.D. Powers & Associates, and other private-sector organizations do for consumer products and service industries; and Underwriters Laboratories actually establishes standards and offers formal certification of products. But instead of a diminution of the FDA's power, responsibilities, and requirements, we have seen quite the opposite.

Massive Civil Litigation: Industry's Worst Nightmare

Health care liability in the United States is governed by a patchwork of different laws in each state and separate rules in the federal court system. Cases litigated in different jurisdictions may operate under different criteria and standards that establish a pharmaceutical manufacturer's liability. Not surprisingly, under this system damage awards can vary widely and may not be even remotely commensurate with the severity of the injury or degree of culpability. Despite a generally high level of

12. The Tufts Center for the Study of Drug Development, *1998 Annual Report* (Boston: Tufts University, 1998), pp. 14–15.

rigor and quality control in the pharmaceutical industry, and intense regulatory scrutiny by the FDA, damage suits against drug and medical device firms have come to exemplify the product liability crisis in the United States. With respect to both the total number of tort liability cases and the share of liability costs relative to industry sales, the pharmaceutical industry has borne a disproportionate share of the liability burden.[13] Since the 1970s, for example, more than a thousand lawsuits have been filed against drug companies on behalf of women who developed vaginal carcinoma because their mothers took the drug diethystilbestrol (DES) to prevent miscarriage during pregnancy; approximately 200,000 women have sued A. H. Robins, alleging damage from the Dalkon Shield intrauterine contraceptive.[14] A particularly troubling aspect of manufacturers' legal liability is a common provision in state laws called joint-and-several liability, which allows enforcement of the entire judgment against any one of the parties found guilty of the tort — with the burden of proof on a manufacturer to show why it could not have caused the alleged damages. This means, for example, that a manufacturer can be ordered to pay the majority of damages even if other parties in the litigation are actually more culpable.

Drug and medical device companies make easy and tempting targets for product liability litigation; they make products that, by their very nature, are intimately involved in life-and-death situations. Furthermore, they are susceptible to claims designed to appeal to the sympathy of jurors amenable to picking the proverbially deep pockets of large companies. Even when no causal relationship between the product and injury or illness in patients is demonstrated, or when the alleged injury is only a trivial side effect listed on the product's label, companies are at risk. For example, from the 1970s through the mid-1980s, almost two

---

13. W. Kip Viscusi, "Regulatory Reform and Liability for Pharmaceuticals and Medical Devices," in Ralph A. Epstein et al., *Advancing Medical Innovation: Health, Safety, and the Role of Government in the 21st Century* (Washington, D.C.: Progress & Freedom Foundation, 1996), pp. 79–102.

14. Deborah R. Hensler and Mark A. Peterson, "Understanding Mass Personal Injury Litigation: A Socio-Legal Analysis," *Brooklyn Law Review* 59B (1993): 961–1063.

thousand lawsuits were filed against Merrell Dow Pharmaceuticals, alleging that the company's drug Bendectin® had caused birth defects in the offspring of women who took the drug to prevent morning sickness during pregnancy.[15] No judgments against the company were ever upheld, but Merrell Dow ultimately discontinued manufacturing the extraordinarily useful drug because it feared that an unreasonable and hostile jury might some day award huge damages.

The most egregious example of damage wrongfully inflicted on a product manufacturer is surely the case of silicone breast implants. Since the first silicone breast implant case went to trial in the 1980s, literally hundreds of thousands of women have filed claims in state courts or through a federal class action settlement. Dozens of studies, conducted by a veritable Who's Who of medical institutions and researchers in the United States and around the world, have failed to find any association between silicone breast implants and disease. Based on this evidence, leading medical organizations, including the American Medical Association, the American College of Rheumatology, and the American Academy of Neurology, have issued statements in favor of the devices. Since 1996, more than three-quarters of the verdicts in silicone breast implant cases have been decided in favor of the defendants, based largely on medical evidence that shows silicone breast implants are not dangerous.[16] The correctness of these verdicts was further supported by an authoritative 1998 report from a federal court-appointed panel of scientists asked to determine whether credible evidence existed that silicone implants are associated with autoimmune diseases, as many plaintiffs had charged.[17] The panel heard testimony from experts on both sides of the issue, consulted its own experts, and examined a large number of documents. They found no convincing scientific evidence that silicone implants cause autoimmune diseases,

15. Marcia Angell, *Science on Trial: The Clash of Medical Evidence and the Law in the Breast Implant Case* (London and New York: W. W. Norton, 1996), p. 75.

16. Ibid., p. 22.

17. John Schwartz, "Scientists Find Little That Links Breast Implants and Disease," *Washington Post*, December 2, 1998, p. A8.

a conclusion shared by the comprehensive study of the safety of silicone implants by the prestigious Institute of Medicine.[18] What has befallen Dow Corning and other manufacturers of breast implants is corporate America's worst nightmare: the virtual annihilation of a successful company through civil lawsuits, in the absence of evidence of either wrongdoing or product defects, or even any association between the product and severe illness. After more than twenty thousand breast implant–related lawsuits, Dow Corning was forced to file for bankruptcy protection.

Experts estimate that our tort system costs Americans $152 billion annually in higher costs for everything from baseball bats and football helmets to automobiles; as much as 20 percent of the price of a stepladder, for example, represents the costs of protection against product liability.[19] That translates to more than $1,000 per household annually in increased product costs. This is not an efficient societal strategy for preventing dangerous products from being sold: The threat of liability suits makes businesses more anxious, to be sure, but the primary issue for them becomes not whether the product is actually safe but how vulnerable the product is to claims of damages. Thus, baseless litigation provides a major disincentive for any company to work on new medical technologies. A corollary is that the lower the profit margin on a product, the more likely it is to be neglected or abandoned by prospective manufacturers, no matter how useful or badly needed it may be.

The fear of litigation is justified. DuPont once supplied Teflon to a small company, Vitek, that used it to make jaw implants. When problems were found with the implants, Vitek declared bankruptcy and the injured patients sued DuPont. Although the courts have generally ruled in the company's favor, DuPont has spent more than $40 million defending itself against the suits, far more than the profit on the few cents'

18. Stuart Bondurant, Virginia Ernster, and Roger Herdman, eds., *Safety of Silicone Breast Implants* (Washington, D.C.: Committee on the Safety of Silicone Breast Implants, Institute of Medicine, National Academy Press, 1999).

19. Stephen Gold, "Step Ladders and Lawsuits," *Washington Times*, November 21, 1997, p. A23.

worth of Teflon in each implant.[20] Such experiences engender a fear of liability suits that can affect the supply of raw materials for pharmaceuticals, leading to product shortages, steep price increases, and even the complete disappearance of critical medical products. More than a dozen major suppliers of raw materials have halted sales to U.S. manufacturers of medical devices—which are typically small, cash-strapped companies—because the risk of litigation far outweighs the benefits of selling these materials.[21] For example, when a supplier of raw materials stopped shipments to the Guidant Corporation in 1994 because of liability concerns, Guidant was forced to take an angioplasty product off the market and then spent millions of dollars and eight man-years of labor recertifying the replacement product.[22]

Vaccines offer another dramatic example of the chilling effect of liability concerns on investment decisions. Because vaccines are administered to large numbers of healthy people, adverse reactions are both more noticeable and of greater concern (especially if they are frequent or severe) than such reactions to therapeutic drugs. Between 1966 and 1977, half of all private vaccine manufacturers stopped making and distributing vaccines, largely because of liability concerns. More recently, a major biotech firm declined to develop an AIDS vaccine because of liability concerns, and another, for the same reasons, withdrew from clinical trials a vaccine that might have prevented the transmission of HIV from infected mothers to their unborn children.

20. Angell, *Science on Trial*, p. 84.
21. Jill Bratina, Ketchum Public Relations, Inc., Washington, D.C., personal communication.
22. Ibid.

3

Reforming the
Current System

Unhappily, the "gold standard" of FDA regulation is fool's gold. By making drug approval more and more difficult, politicized, and arbitrary, by obstructing instead of facilitating and guiding the process, the FDA has become an untrustworthy guardian of public health.

The United States remains in the forefront of drug discovery and development only by dint of a combination of American ingenuity, prodigious investment, technological prowess, and the flexibility to perform clinical trials abroad—outside the jurisdiction of the FDA. However, the opportunity costs of excessive regulation are high, and when other factors that confound drug development are also considered, it is remarkable that the nation has not already relinquished its leadership position. The increased prominence of nontraditional obstacles facing drug companies, including product liability suits and new extragovernmental standards, have added to the burdens imposed by highly risk-averse federal regulation. These challenges to the bottom line, discussed in the previous chapter, have driven the dramatic consolidation of the research-based industry during the past decade. In addition, since the return on investment to the innovative manufacturer has fallen and become more uncertain, more resources are being channeled into less regulated channels—for example, nonresearch and development areas such as sales.

At the same time, U.S. companies are concentrating more of their research and development efforts abroad in countries where the regulatory burden is not as onerous. Comparing drug review in five countries, Rawson et al. noted that from 1992 to 1995, mean approval times in the United States were significantly longer than those in the United Kingdom and Sweden and the same as those in Australia.[1] The effects are striking: In the area of anticancer drugs, for example, during the 1960s cancer patients in the United States had more therapeutic agents available to them than did patients in the United Kingdom, Germany, France, or Japan. Now, in contrast, patients in the United States have fewer choices available than in those countries.

Many practicing physicians are highly critical of the FDA. In a 1995 survey of clinical oncologists conducted by the Competitive Enterprise Institute (CEI), nearly two-thirds of respondents agreed that the FDA "hurt their ability to give the best possible care to a patient on at least one occasion," and over one in ten said this happened "frequently."[2] Three-quarters of respondents "opposed FDA restrictions on off-label information," and 60 percent indicated that those restrictions made their job more difficult. Similar results were obtained in a subsequent CEI survey of cardiologists, published in 1996. Half maintained that FDA regulations prevented them from using promising new drugs or medical devices, 71 percent responded that the FDA's approval process hurt their ability to give patients the best care, and 57 percent expressed the belief that unnecessary delays in product approval by the FDA actually cost lives.[3] Similarly, 80 percent of the respondents to a 1998

1. Nigel S. B. Rawson et al., "Drug Review in Canada: A Comparison with Australia, Sweden, the United Kingdom, and the United States," *Drug Information Journal* 32 (1998): 1133–41.

2. Competitive Enterprise Institute, *A National Survey of Oncologists regarding the Food and Drug Administration* (Washington, D.C.: Competitive Enterprise Institute, August 1995).

3. Competitive Enterprise Institute, *A National Survey of Cardiologists regarding the Food and Drug Administration* (Washington, D.C.: Competitive Enterprise Institute, July 1996).

CEI survey of neurologists and neurosurgeons said the FDA process hurt their ability to treat patients.[4] Finally, 64 percent of respondents to a 1999 survey of emergency room physicians said the FDA is too slow in approving new drugs and devices, and 51 percent maintained that existing pharmaceutical regulation actually costs patients' lives.[5] So much for FDA regulation as the world's gold standard.

The FDA's oversight of the development and use of pharmaceuticals has changed American industrial innovation in subtle ways. Concerns about costs and projected returns on investment increasingly drive drug development. Owing to the high costs and uncertain outcome of seeking government approval for product testing and marketing, research tends to focus on lower-risk research projects that are unlikely to encounter significant regulatory problems and are intended for potentially large patient populations. The high costs of approval, coupled with an imperfect capital market, also act to keep potential entrants out of the industry. Putting it another way, via several mechanisms, including the widespread consolidation of the drug industry and fewer products overall in the research and development pipeline, overregulation and its attendant costs, lead to diminished competition. However, following several waves of mergers in the industry, the ever-bigger drug manufacturers' evermore formidable regulatory affairs apparatuses have become comfortable with the present system. Some companies seem happy to take on the competition not on the merits of research and development but at negotiating their way through the regulatory maze. This jaded outlook may explain some of the industry's apathy toward congressional reform of the FDA during the 1990s (chapter 4).[6]

4. Competitive Enterprise Institute, *A National Survey of Neurologists and Neurosurgeons regarding the Food and Drug Administration* (Washington, D.C.: Competitive Enterprise Institute, October 1998).

5. Competitive Enterprise Institute, *A National Survey of Emergency Room Physicians regarding the Food and Drug Administration* (Washington, D.C.: Competitive Enterprise Institute, October 1999).

6. Henry I. Miller, "Failed FDA Reform," *Regulation* 21 (1998): 24–30.

"Europe's FDA":
Competition and Outside Review Make It Work

Comparable regulatory agencies in other countries employ other approaches to the oversight of pharmaceutical development, and comparisons to the FDA can be instructive. The experience abroad may, in fact, hold the key to understanding how oversight in the United States might be revised and improved. Data from European countries such as the United Kingdom, Sweden, and Germany and from the European Union's evolving system of regulation suggest that the U.S. approval process is highly inefficient and that the institutions performing drug and device review and approval in certain other countries have more successfully balanced assurance of product safety and efficacy, innovation, and medical progress.[7]

Consider, for example, the supranational equivalent of the FDA, the centralized European Agency for the Evaluation of Medicinal Products (EMEA), headquartered in London. The EMEA is lean, efficient, surprisingly unbureaucratic, and remarkably well regarded by the drug industry. Established in 1995, it coordinates the scientific resources of the individual drug regulatory agencies of the nations of the European Union, each of which is itself analogous to the U.S. FDA. Dual systems exist for drug evaluation and approval in the European Union. The EMEA offers a centralized procedure, compulsory for biotechnology and optional for other innovative new products. That mechanism in effect competes with a decentralized procedure that is based on "mutual recognition of national authorizations," or reciprocity among the regulatory systems in each of the member countries.[8] Reciprocity means the extension of one nation's marketing approval to one or more other

7. Kenneth I. Kaitin and Jeffrey S. Brown, "A Drug Lag Update," in Kenneth I. Kaitin, ed., "White Paper on Four Areas of Relevance to New Drug Development and Review in the United States," *Drug Information Journal* 29 (1995): 355–424.

8. Elaine M. Healy and Kenneth I. Kaitin, "The European Agency for the Evaluation of Medicinal Products' Centralized Procedure for Product Approval: Current Status," *Drug Information Journal* 33 (1999): 969–77.

members of the European Union. This competition engenders administrative and other efficiencies and has been an important factor in the EMEA's success. Another, more subtle level of competition in European drug evaluation is the EMEA's ability to choose reviewers from a multinational pool of 2,300 available experts. This means that, with time, the overall level of expertise tends to rise; incompetent, excessively slow, or adversarial reviewers simply don't get work and are eliminated. (At the FDA, by contrast, reviews are performed in-house, and civil service rules prevent anyone—even those who are chronically incompetent or adversarial—from being fired; agency managers have to make do with what they have.)

In the centralized procedure, applications for marketing approval are submitted directly to the EMEA in London. At the conclusion of a 210-day evaluation by the product's scientific committee, which is composed of several experts drawn from the EMEA's stable of reviewers throughout Europe, its opinion is transmitted to the European Commission. After an additional 90 days, the commission issues a single market authorization that applies to the whole European Union.[9] Although it is difficult to compare the efficiency of the EMEA directly to that of the U.S. FDA, the average period of clinical testing is substantially longer in the United States, and data are available that indicate how differently the agencies are perceived by their corporate clients. In a 1997 survey of the interactions between drug companies and the FDA conducted by researchers at the University of California at San Diego,[10] 78 percent of companies that responded said poor "clarity of data requests" from the agency had "impeded or stopped" the development of their products. In 62 percent, personnel turnover at the FDA had impeded or stopped the review process. In 40 percent, limitations in the FDA reviewers' technical knowledge had slowed the progress of a product. At the same time, an anonymous survey by the EMEA of its own

9. Ibid.
10. California Health Care Institute and Ernst & Young, *Exporting an Industry: The Impact of FDA Regulation on California's Biomedical Industry* (San Diego: California Health Care Institute and Ernst & Young, 1996).

applicants found that 33 percent were very satisfied, 61 percent were satisfied, and 6 percent were dissatisfied.[11] Moreover, as of 1999, according to Healy and Kaitin, the majority of the marketing authorizations granted by the EMEA were for products whose review through this mechanism was optional, implying a high level of industry satisfaction with the centralized procedure.[12]

The EMEA's mean processing time was 207 days for marketing applications *received* in 1997, whereas the FDA required 460 days for the marketing approvals that were *announced* in 1997. The FDA is in fact even slower than the comparison suggests because the way the FDA reports data makes its numbers appear more favorable than they are; that is, reporting only the approvals *announced* in 1997 tends to minimize the statistical impact of applications languishing unapproved for long periods.

The regulatory philosophies of the EMEA and FDA are very different. The EMEA focuses narrowly on performing "high quality evaluation of medicinal products," monitoring product safety, offering advice on research and development programs, and providing "useful and clear information to users and health professionals," according to its mission statement.[13] It relies on summary reports supplied by the sponsor, carefully tracks and publicizes indicators of its own performance, and is perceived as client-friendly. The FDA, by contrast, is compliance-oriented, comports itself like a police agency—it actually has armed inspectors—and frequently treats drug companies like adversaries (*vide infra*). Rather than relying on summary reports supplied by the sponsor, the FDA's review typically involves arduous reanalysis of the sponsor's original raw data.

---

11. Fernand Sauer, European Agency for the Evaluation of Medicinal Products, personal communication.

12. Elaine M. Healy and Kenneth I. Kaitin, "The European Agency for the Evaluation of Medicinal Products' Centralized Procedure for Product Approval: Current Status." *Drug Information Journal* 33 (1999): 969–78.

13. The European Agency for the Evaluation of Medicinal Products (EMEA), *Work Programme 1998–99* (London: EMEA, 1998).

An FDA out of Control

One of economist Milton Friedman's best-known observations is that individuals and organizations usually act in ways that favor their own self-interest. Certainly the policies and product decisions of the FDA and other regulatory agencies confirm the truth of that insight. Civil servants and political appointees spend a lot of time and energy thinking about simply staying out of trouble and avoiding adverse publicity, and this, combined with the arbitrariness and lack of accountability of the current system, encourages various kinds of behavior that are inimical to the public interest. For example, special interest groups try to gain advantage from the FDA by special pleading; individuals have increasingly found that by forming aggressive advocacy groups—as patients suffering from AIDS have done—they can force the FDA to expedite approval of medications to treat their afflictions. Regulators tend to favor certain groups solely because of their skillful application of political pressure and manipulation of the media. This means that other medications with greater public health impact but less well-organized constituencies might receive less than equal treatment. Such capriciousness and vulnerability to pressure reflect the way that the current system is gamed. Regulators do what is in their own self-interest—in this case, avoiding a thrashing on the evening news for foot-dragging on certain approvals—instead of what is in the public interest.

Another aspect of self-interest pertains to regulators' fear of being perceived as too eager to approve new products. In the early 1980s, when I headed the team at the FDA that was reviewing the NDA for recombinant human insulin, the first drug made with gene-splicing techniques, we were ready to recommend approval a mere four months after the application was submitted (at a time when the average time for NDA review was more than two and a half years). With quintessential bureaucratic reasoning, my supervisor refused to sign off on the approval—even though he agreed that the data provided compelling evidence of the drug's safety and effectiveness. "If anything goes wrong," he argued "think how bad it will look that we approved the drug so quickly." (When the supervisor went on vacation, I convinced his boss to sign off on the approval.) The supervisor was more concerned with not looking bad in case of an unforeseen mishap than with getting an important new product to patients who needed it. This system lacks predictability, fairness, and integrity, but given the existing incentives and disincentives, risks and rewards, at the FDA, an official's decision to put self-interest above the public interest is hardly surprising. However, as former FDA commissioner Donald Kennedy has observed, individual regulators are not wholly blameworthy for conforming to a system that rewards certain dubious patterns of decision making.

Regulatory officials' tendency to maximize their self-interest must be seen in light of the marked asymmetry between the two basic kinds of mistaken decisions that a drug regulator can make: (1) a harmful product is approved for marketing, a *type 1* error in the parlance of risk assessment, or (2) a useful product that treats or prevents disease is rejected, delayed, never achieves marketing approval or is inappropriately withdrawn from the market, a *type 2* error. In other words, a regulator commits a type 1 error by permitting something harmful to happen and a type 2 error by preventing something beneficial from becoming available. Both situations have negative consequences for the public, but the outcomes for the regulator are very different.

A classic type 1 error (or what was perceived as a type 1 error, which is much the same thing) was the FDA's approval in 1976 of the swine flu vaccine. Although the vaccine was effective at preventing influenza (of a strain that, ironically, did not cause an epidemic), it had a major side effect that was unknown at the time of approval: temporary paralysis from Guillain-Barré Syndrome in a small number of patients. This kind of mistake is highly visible and has immediate consequences—the media pounces, the public denounces, and Congress pronounces. Both the developers of the product and the regulators who allowed it to be marketed are excoriated and punished in modern-day pillories: congressional hearings, television news magazines, and newspaper editorials. Because a regulatory official's career might be damaged irreparably by his good faith but mistaken approval of a high-profile product, decisions are often made defensively—in other words, to avoid type 1 errors at any cost. This brings to mind, of course, the review of human insulin described above where the supervisor delayed the approval, not because of any concerns about the quality of the product or the data supporting its approval but only because it would "look bad" if a problem ultimately occurred in a quickly approved drug. This predilection, or pressure, toward commission of type 2 errors is not the way the system is supposed to operate. Lifetime tenure for civil servants—which itself exacts costs—is supposed to free regulators to consider only the public interest as they render decisions. Instead, it has given us the worst of both worlds: On the one hand, it has become virtually impossible to remove incompetent or adversarial federal civil servants; on the other, we are forced to live with decision making by federal officials that is frequently influenced by perceived risks to their careers.

Type 2 errors in the form of unreasonable governmental require-ments and decisions can delay the marketing of a new product, lessen competition to produce it, and inflate its ultimate price. They can even prevent marketing of a product entirely. Consider, again, the FDA's precipitate and inappropriate response to the 1999 death of a patient in a University of Pennsylvania gene-therapy trial for a genetic disease. Within a few months, the FDA had clamped several other kinds of unwarranted controls on gene-therapy investigators, including the re-quirement for all sponsors of gene-therapy products to submit to the agency substantial additional information—not only about the trials themselves but also about animal studies and materials that may have been intended for use in clinical trials but were not so used for one reason or another. Although the cause of the incident had not been identified, and the product class (a preparation of a desired gene, en-cased in an enfeebled adenovirus) had been used in a large number of patients with no fatalities, and serious side effects in only a small per-centage of patients, the FDA reacted disproportionately. The agency not only stopped the trial in which the fatality occurred and all the other gene-therapy studies at the same university but also halted similar stud-ies at other universities as well as experiments using adenovirus being conducted by drug company Schering-Plough—one for the treatment of liver cancer, the other for colorectal cancer that had metastasized to the liver.[14] In these ways, and by publicly excoriating and humiliating the researchers involved (and halting experiments of theirs that did not even involve adenovirus), the FDA cast a pall over the entire field of gene therapy.[15]

Although they can dramatically compromise public health, type 2 errors caused by a regulator's poor judgment, timidity, or anxiety seldom gain public attention. Usually, only the company that makes the product is likely to be aware. Likewise, if the regulator's mistake precipitates a corporate decision to abandon the product, cause and effect are seldom connected in the public mind. There may be no direct evidence of the lost benefits or of the culpability of regulatory officials. Exceptions exist, of course. A few activists, such as the AIDS advocacy groups that closely monitor the FDA, scrutinize agency review of certain products and aggressively publicize type 2 errors. Congressional oversight should provide a check on regulators' performance, but only rarely does it focus on their type 2 errors (type 1 errors make for more exciting hearings, with injured patients prominently featured). Even when such mistakes are exposed, regulators frequently defend type 2 errors as erring on the side of caution, as they did in the Pennsylvania gene therapy case. Too often this euphemism is accepted uncritically by legislators, the media, and the public, and our system of pharmaceutical oversight becomes progressively less relevant to the public interest. Several examples of FDA policies that illustrate the congruence between regulators' type 2 errors and the agency's inexorable expansion into new areas are discussed below in the sections on the FDA's censorship of medical articles, new rules for reporting side effects, and requirements for pediatric testing of drugs.

The self-interest of individual officials and the FDA as a whole pro-

14. Henry I. Miller, "Ill-advised Response to a Tragedy," *Financial Times*, January 14, 2000, p. 19.
15. Henry I. Miller, "Gene Therapy's Trials and Tribulations," *The Scientist*, February 7, 2000, p. 16.

foundly affects the agency's receptivity to and the fate of regulatory reform. During the past thirty years, agency officials have received no bouquets from Congress or the public for attempts to decrease regulatory mandates, improve efficiency, and reduce requirements. Quite the opposite—the rewards have gone to those who have succeeded in expanding their responsibilities, budgets, and empires. Moreover, busywork, such as the creation and evaluation of milestones in performance plans, has become a major industry within the FDA.

More than a hundred studies, inquiries, and congressional hearings have documented the negative impacts of the existing system.[16] According to a report from the Tufts Center for the Study of Drug Development, "the regulatory activities of the FDA may constitute the most thoroughly investigated and studied program of government regulation in history."[17] As early as 1955, the report of the Hoover Commission's Task Force on Federal Medical Services found that the FDA was outmoded, used punitive methods, and had inadequate staff.[18] In 1966, the Miles Committee (reporting to Secretary of Health, Education and Welfare John W. Gardner) described the need for improved management and greater scientific competence at the agency.[19] In 1973 the President's Science Advisory Committee concluded that U.S. regulations should be modified "to ensure that no important new entity introduced into selected foreign countries during the previous year failed to become available in the United States."[20] Three years later, the President's Biomedical Panel concluded that the FDA was a "formidable

16. Kenneth I. Kaitin, ed., executive summary of "White Paper on Four Areas of Relevance to New Drug Development and Review in the United States," *Drug Information Journal* 29 (1995): 357–59.

17. Peter Barton Hutt, "Investigations and Reports respecting FDA Regulation of New Drugs (Part I)," *Clinical Pharmacology and Therapeutics* 33 (1987): 537.

18. Sheila R. Shulman, Peg Hewitt, and Michael Manocchia, "Studies and Inquiries into the FDA Regulatory Process: A Historical Perspective," *Drug Information Journal* (1995): 385–413.

19. Ibid.

20. *Report of the Panel on Chemicals and Health of the President's Science Advisory Committee* (Washington, D.C.: Science and Technology Policy Office, National Science Foundation, 1973), p. 113.

roadblock" and that the agency's delays and costs to drug development constituted a "hazard to public health."[21] Between 1982 and 1992 alone, the activities and policies of the FDA were the subject of nine major reports or sets of recommendations from government sources and independent commissions;[22] in 1982, for example, the Hayes Task Force (reporting to the Office of Management and Budget, via Secretary of Health and Human Services Richard S. Schweiker) made a number of recommendations related to New Drug Applications, including reducing the bulk of NDA submissions, streamlining the NDA format, greater use of foreign data, and greater adherence by the FDA to meeting the 180-day statutory time limit for review.[23] The reports of these studies, however, just seem to get filed away and forgotten.

Of particular relevance to the proposal made in this volume is the fact that at least twenty-nine independent studies have produced recommendations that would transfer some tasks performed internally by the FDA to outside experts. Other oft-repeated recommendations include overarching management and structural reforms and changes in the FDA's culture that would redress regulators' single-minded avoidance of type 1 errors (although it has seldom been stated in those terms). The following call for broader and more meaningful cost-benefit analysis, and for a change in the incentives and disincentives to drug regulators, for example, came from Robert B. Helms at a 1981 conference on the development and oversight of drugs:

> The legislative mandate to FDA officials should . . . be reconsidered: they should not be forced into the inefficient strategy of seeking zero risk. A common myth in the regulatory reform debate is that regulation may be improved simply by replacing the present regulators with better qualified ones. Most serious analysts of drug regulation, however, have not blamed the poor performance of the FDA on the people as much as on

21. "Report of the President's Biomedical Research Panel, Appendix A," U.S. Department of Health, Education and Welfare publication (OS) 76-50, 1976, pp. 19–21.

22. Sheila R. Shulman, Peg Hewitt, and Michael Manocchia, "Studies and Inquiries into the FDA Regulatory Process."

23. Ibid.

the incentives established by the legislation. . . . The trouble is that Congress has given the FDA and other health and safety regulatory agencies a single mandate to reduce risk to consumers. Some analysts feel that this bias in favor of reducing risk, regardless of the cost of forgone benefits, should be substantially changed: the mandate should also consider the costs of agency decisions and, in the case of drugs, the potential benefits of new drugs to patients.[24]

Helms is correct that meaningful change requires congressional action, but Congress's sporadic interest in drug regulation has usually taken the form of spurious, politically motivated concerns about *under-regulation*. The bottom line is that Congress's failure to carry out its oversight and legislative responsibilities has permitted the problems to become progressively worse and more entrenched. We face a situation in which neither the FDA nor Congress possesses sufficient commitment to the public interest to undertake true reform. Their failures are explored in the next chapter.

24. Robert B. Helms, ed., editor's preface to *Drugs and Health: Economic Issues and Policy Objectives* (Washington D.C.: American Enterprise Institute for Public Policy Research, 1981), xxiv–xxv.

4

The Failure of
Self-Reform and
Congressional Reform

Self-Reform: The Fox in the Henhouse

Like most regulatory agencies, the FDA tries to conciliate its congressional and executive branch masters by making public pronouncements that are likely to mollify its critics of the moment. But within the current system, regulators' self-interest is not served by the implementation of meaningful change, so real reform is never accomplished. Instead, boxes on the organizational chart are arranged and rearranged, added and eliminated; names of entities are changed (and then changed back); and various pilot programs come and go. FDA managers avidly craft and meet new performance milestones, but there is little impact on the bottom line of timely patients' access to new therapies. Often the FDA simply codifies or promotes changes that have already evolved or been implemented. For example, in a grandly titled 1995 press release, "Reinventing Drug and Medical Device Regulation," the FDA announced a lengthy list of reforms,[1] but none had more than minimal impact and most were already well within the agency's practices or discretion.[2] Robert Yetter, associate director for policy at the FDA's Center for

1. Food and Drug Administration, "Reinventing Drug and Medical Device Regulation" (press release, April 6, 1995).
2. Henry I. Miller, "With FDA You Get Indigestion," *San Jose Mercury News*, May 25, 1995, 7B.

Biologics Evaluation and Research, admitted as much at a conference sponsored by the Food and Drug Law Institute in July 1999. When asked to point out the single most important aspect of the 1997 FDA Modernization Act (FDAMA), that was supposedly the most significant FDA reform in three decades, Yetter answered, "It put into law many things that FDA was already doing." Now that's a ringing endorsement! It's also the full extent of progressive thinking we can expect from the FDA. The agency is averse to radical change and to any diminution of its responsibilities. As described in the next two sections, what the agency touts as reform does not get drugs to patients any more rapidly or any more cheaply. It has more to do with public relations than public health.

Biological Drugs

In 1996, the FDA announced that it would modernize and streamline the oversight of a class of therapeutic products called biological drugs, or biologicals, which includes blood and blood products, vaccines, derivatives of natural substances for treating allergies, extracts of living cells, and most products of the new biotechnology.[3] Since the 1902 act that ushered in consumer product regulation, these products had been approached by regulators differently from others because the difficulty in producing biologicals meant that they were often impure compared to other drugs. Also biologicals tended to be poorly characterized and inconsistent; one batch might contain 2 percent of the active substance and another, 4 percent, with widely varying amounts of other constituents. Because it was difficult to demonstrate that each batch met specified standards of purity and potency, two discrete kinds of approvals were required. The FDA granted marketing approval for the product itself, which had to be safe and effective, and the agency licensed the

---

3. Food and Drug Administration, "Elimination of Establishment License Application for Specified Biotechnology and Specified Synthetic Biological Products," *Federal Register* 61 (May 14, 1996): 24227–33.

manufacturing establishment, which had to show proof of adequate control over and rigor in production. The FDA also certified samples from every production batch.

Nonbiological drugs are traditionally smaller, simpler, chemically synthesized molecules that can be purified and characterized much more easily than biologicals. In contrast to biologicals, neither licensing of the manufacturing facility nor batch certification for those products was required.

Advances in technology over the past two decades have blurred the distinction between biological and other drugs. The majority of biologicals—particularly those made with the techniques of the new biotechnology such as recombinant DNA, or gene splicing—are now highly purified, well-characterized preparations that can be regulated the same as other drugs. Biologicals' manufacturing facilities continued to be certified, but in practice the process was not very different from the inspections performed on the plants that make nonbiological drugs. The FDA's 1995 policy change enabled biologicals that were "well characterized biotechnology products" to be regulated as though they were nonbiological drugs. For this subset of biotechnology products, the requirements for licensing the manufacturing facility and for batch certification were eliminated. (And in a bury-the-bone, dig-up-the-bone exercise to make the regulatory change seem more substantial, the agency convened industry-FDA conferences for the purpose of defining the term "well characterized.")

Although this evolution of policy was positive, it was hardly new. Nor was it likely to have much impact, especially in view of the fact that only about two dozen biotechnology-derived biologicals were approved by the FDA during all of the 1990s. However, in Section 123 of the 1997 FDA Modernization Act (*vide infra*), Congress saw fit to eliminate the requirement for sponsors of biological drugs to obtain separate product and establishment licenses (and the FDA subsequently issued new regulations that require only the single Biologics License Application). This illustrates perfectly FDA official Robert Yetter's characterization, above, of FDAMA as merely codifying what the agency was already doing.

Surrogate End Points

A more disingenuous sample of pseudoreform occurred on March 29, 1996, the very day after three FDA reform bills were introduced in the House of Representatives. President Bill Clinton, Vice President Al Gore, Health and Human Services secretary Donna Shalala, and then FDA commissioner David Kessler announced with great hoopla that thenceforth the FDA would permit the use of so-called surrogate end points to speed up the process of cancer-drug development.[4] Specifically, they asserted that "it is appropriate to utilize objective evidence of tumor shrinkage as a basis for approval, allowing additional evidence of increased survival and/or improved quality of life associated with that therapy to be demonstrated later."[5]

In order to appreciate that there was nothing at all new about this approach to assessing a drug's efficacy, some background on surrogate end points is necessary. As in the example of the second-generation hepatitis B vaccine described in chapter 2, the ultimate indicator of the clinical benefit of a drug is an unambiguously positive outcome such as survival or the complete disappearance of disease, but frequently these are difficult and expensive to demonstrate as the end point of clinical trials. Therefore, physicians and others involved in clinical testing, including the FDA, have over several decades come to accept appropriate surrogates as measures of a disease's amelioration, regression, or prevention. For drugs that lower blood pressure or serum cholesterol, for example, the FDA no longer requires a demonstration that treatment actually increases survival or reduces the incidence of heart attacks and stroke: significant improvement of "the numbers"—that is,

---

4. William J. Clinton and Albert Gore Jr., *Reinventing the Regulation of Cancer Drugs: Accelerating Approval and Expanding Access*, National Performance Review (Washington, D.C.: White House, March 1996).
    5. Ibid.

lowering of blood pressure or of cholesterol or an improvement in the pattern of serum lipids (a greater proportion of "good" lipids)—along with documentation of safety are sufficient. If clinical trials of every new cholesterol-lowering agent and blood pressure drug were still required to demonstrate improvement in the ultimate end points of increased survival or fewer heart attacks, the cost of developing those drugs would be dramatically and unnecessarily increased. Surrogate end points in some form already had been used for decades before the Clinton-Gore-Shalala-Kessler announcement. More to the point, starting in 1991, as a result of reforms stimulated by President George Bush's Council on Competitiveness, the FDA had formally adopted (at least in theory) a policy of using flexibility in the current statute to develop and adopt surrogate end points whenever possible as a measure of the efficacy of drugs used to treat life-threatening diseases.[6] Thus, the Clinton administration was touting as a major reform what was already official FDA policy. In itself, this misrepresentation is not a grave transgression, nor can patients be said to have been injured directly or indirectly by it. But it does illustrate the government's cynical approach to educating the public about drug regulation, and it shows how politicized the procedures and policies of the nation's foremost regulatory agency have become.

Congressional Reform:
Where There's No Will, There's No Way

If the FDA cannot reform itself it is up to Congress to impose reform, something it has lacked the will to do. The one serious attempt in recent decades, the sweeping Drugs and Biological Products Reform Act of 1996, HR 3199, went down to ignominious defeat.[7] HR 3199 would

6. President's Council on Competitiveness, *Improving the Nation's Drug Approval Process* (Washington, D.C.: White House, November 1991) (fact sheet).

7. Drug and Biological Products Reform Act of 1996, HR 3199, introduced into the 104th Congress, 2d Session.

have allowed the FDA in many cases to dispense with the requirement that manufacturers turn over voluminous raw data from clinical trials. Manufacturers instead would have delivered condensed, tabulated, or summarized data—just as they do now in submissions to the FDA's foreign counterparts—but the agency would have retained access to additional material when it was needed. This legislation would also have established a new, more liberal approval standard for drugs intended to treat any "serious or life-threatening" condition.[8] Like the then current standard for AIDS drugs, the new criterion would have allowed easier access by patients with other illnesses to a drug when there is "a reasonable likelihood that the drug will be effective in a significant number of patients and that the risk from the drug is no greater than the risk from the condition."[9] That commonsense, humane principle would have extended to patients with diseases like stroke, multiple sclerosis, Alzheimer's disease, emphysema, crippling arthritis, and heart failure the benefits reserved for those with AIDS.

The bill would have ameliorated to a large extent the FDA's censorship of scientific and medical information concerning off-label uses (not yet approved uses of a drug sanctioned for another purpose) by permitting the legitimate dissemination of information about unapproved uses to health professionals and the public via textbooks and articles from peer-reviewed journals. It would also have permitted retrospective evidence from clinical research to be used for approval of additional, off-label uses of drugs already on the market. Expensive and time-consuming new studies are normally required for new uses even when some data from the original tests are perfectly adequate. Such a reform would have cut down both on the time and on the costs involved in securing FDA approval for additional uses of drugs.

The legislation's most significant reform—echoing proposals made by my coauthors and myself earlier that same year in the Progress &

8. Ibid., Section 5.
9. Ibid.

Freedom Foundation's study *Advancing Medical Innovation*[10] —would have introduced nongovernmental alternatives to some FDA oversight. Under its provisions, pharmaceutical manufacturers could have opted for product review by FDA-accredited nongovernmental organizations. Each of these institutions would have been subject to periodic FDA audits, and strict requirements backed by civil and criminal sanctions would have assured the confidentiality of data and the absence of conflicts of interest. Alternatively, the manufacturer could have opted for review by the FDA; in all cases the agency would have retained the responsibility for final sign-off of marketing approvals. Of course, permitting the FDA to retain sign-off on its competitors' recommendations is rather like giving Coca Cola the right to sign off on Pepsi taste tests. Despite such shortcomings, had it been enacted, the bill would have been a significant step toward loosening the FDA's monopoly grip.

The fate met by HR 3199 is instructive. The FDA and its supporters in the Clinton administration saw the legislation as a threat to the federal government's regulatory hegemony, and they pulled out all the stops to defeat it. Then Assistant Secretary of Health and Human Services Phil Lee dismissed the bill and anything resembling it as nothing more than veto bait. Then FDA commissioner David Kessler registered the FDA's opposition to the House bill in a nine-page statement, "The Impact of the House FDA Reform Proposals,"[11] that was remarkable for revealing the lengths to which an agency head will go to protect the status quo. Kessler asserted that the "FDA would be forced to approve new drugs using summaries of safety data prepared by drug companies." Untrue. The bill merely clarified that rather than reviewing the voluminous raw data from clinical trials, often running to hundreds of thousands of

---

10. Henry I. Miller and William M. Wardell, "Therapeutic Drugs and Biologics," in Ralph A. Epstein et al., *Advancing Medical Innovation: Health, Safety, and the Role of Government in the 21st Century* (Washington, D.C.: Progress & Freedom Foundation, 1996), pp. 79–102.

11. Food and Drug Administration, *The Impact of the House FDA Reform Proposals* (Washington, D.C.: Food and Drug Administration, 1996) (background paper).

pages, condensed, tabulated, or summarized data often would be adequate. (As noted above, agency reviewers would have retained access to additional materials as well; all that would have been required was a request by an FDA supervisory official.) To make his case, Kessler cited the example of a drug called Dilevalol®, which he said was approved in Japan, Portugal, and England on the basis of data summaries. Americans, he said, were spared morbidity and mortality because "the FDA medical reviewer noted in the raw data evidence that some patients had severe liver injury." Another untruth. The record shows it was the *manufacturer*, Schering-Plough, that identified the toxicity and ultimately withdrew the application for U.S. approval.[12] Kessler claimed that the legislation would weaken the effectiveness standard for drugs and that the FDA would be forced to approve a new use for a drug on the bases of "anecdotal evidence of effectiveness" and "common use by physicians (with no objective evidence)." The price, he concluded, would be "the unnecessary pain and suffering patients would undergo until they were given an effective treatment." These are more distortions of the truth. The reality is that, as described in chapter 3, the FDA's policies have made life progressively more dangerous for patients and difficult for physicians.

Because of the Clinton administration's vehement opposition to HR 3199 and the threat of a presidential veto, Congress abandoned it. This was a significant loss, given the consensus within the scientific and public policy community that reform was badly needed. Neither before nor since has Congress tackled FDA reform so aggressively, although the agency's policies and performance have begged for it. The legislation that eventually passed in the next congressional session was meager and disappointing.

When the 105th Congress resurrected regulatory reform in 1996–1997, reformers had a succulent carrot to dangle before officials in the Clinton administration: FDA user fees—a generally popular supple-

---

12. Alex R. Giaquinto, letter to House Commerce Committee from Schering-Plough Research Institute, May 14, 1996.

ment to the congressional appropriation, that garnered approximately $100 million annually from industry to help the FDA expedite the approval of new medicines. The authorization for the user fees was set to expire on October 1, 1997, and the desire to obtain another five-year reauthorization provided a strong incentive for the Clinton administration to accept meaningful reforms. However, the 1997 FDA Modernization Act, passed on November 9 and signed by President Clinton on November 20, was the moral equivalent of the proverbial elephant laboring to bring forth a mouse. (Perhaps the metaphor should be an elephant laboring to bring forth a donkey, given the mascots of our two major political parties and the fact that what emerged from the Republican-controlled Congress was a bill dictated and written by Democrats.) To the uninitiated, the sheer volume of the legislation and its laundry list of provisions offer the impression of substance, which was precisely Congress's intent. As discussed below, however, it lacks any major or fundamental reforms.

Section 903(b) of the law adds to the FDA's mission the obligation for "promptly and efficiently reviewing clinical research" and making decisions "in a timely manner." Mission statements alone, however, do not create reform any more than politicians' pronouncements represent reality, and it is naive to think that this symbolism will alter the agency's four-decade-old mind-set of aversion to product and career risks. This section, as well as section 803(c)(3), also requires the FDA to meet with foreign governments and to participate in efforts at international harmonization of regulation. Such requirements are only slightly more than symbolic; legislation can't dictate cooperation, just a presence at the table. The agency has, indeed, reached agreements with its foreign counterparts on issues such as reciprocal recognition of inspections and harmonizing the kinds of information required for certain submissions, but the FDA has been consistently recalcitrant on the pivotal issue of reciprocity of approvals. At one point, when asked by the author how negotiations were progressing, a high-ranking European regulator (who requested anonymity) quipped, "Discussing reciprocity with FDA is like discussing the Thanksgiving menu with the turkeys." Reciprocity of approvals would mean that part of the FDA's review functions would be, in effect, performed gratis by foreign regulators. Such a move would improve the agency's productivity and decrease costs to U.S. taxpayers, but it would also weaken the FDA's monopoly and thus is opposed by the agency.

Section 903(f)(2) of the legislation calls on the FDA to develop a plan for clearing the legendary backlog of products awaiting approval. With this provision, Congress has opened the door to an endless series of demands for additional resources the agency will claim are essential for meeting the required goal. Senior FDA officials have not missed a single public opportunity to "cry poor" since the passage of FDAMA. A related negative effect of the legislation is that it has spawned a major industry of busywork within the FDA—the creation of thousands of arbitrary, bureaucratic milestones that only diverts regulators from the actual work of product review and approval. The magnitude of these activities can be appreciated by examining the portion of the agency's web site devoted to FDAMA at www.fda.gov/opacom/7modact.html (accessed April 7, 2000).

Section 115(a) of the new law permits the FDA to approve a drug for marketing on the basis of a single clinical trial (previous statutory language referred to trials, plural), a change that is entirely symbolic. The FDA easily could have made a case for approval on the basis of a single, definitive, multicenter trial under the earlier language (or simply have asked the drug sponsor to divide the single trial into two, to conform to the language of the statute). But the point is moot. The average number of trials performed to support approval of a new drug is currently approximately seventy (up from thirty two decades ago).[13] Permitting federal regulators to do what they are strongly disinclined to do is unlikely to improve the process of oversight and approval.

Several other sections of the new law codify policies that were already

13. Carl C. Peck, "Drug Development: Improving the Process," *Food & Drug Law Journal* (1997): 163–67.

in place or make inconsequential changes by conferring on the FDA flexibility it had already exercised (similar to the Clinton administration's strategy of "recycling" extant policies, discussed above). For example, Section 124 provides that a drug manufactured in a pilot or other small-scale facility can be used to establish safety and effectiveness for the purpose of approval before scale-up to a full-scale manufacturing facility. But this was already permitted by the FDA. Section 123 eliminates the requirement for separate product and establishment licenses for biological drugs (discussed above), a provision that is desirable but inconsequential because the FDA had already eliminated the important distinctions between biological and other drugs. These kinds of statutory changes attempted to convey the impression of a lengthy list of genuine improvements but actually did little to improve on the status quo.

Section 401 of the legislation ostensibly offers drug companies greater latitude in supplying scientifically sound information to doctors and other health professionals about the off-label uses of prescription drugs, a reform that was sorely needed. Yet it falls far short of what could have been done and what had been proposed in HR 3199 (discussed above). Moreover, the minor improvement wrought by FDAMA on this issue comes at a high price. A manufacturer can disseminate information to health professionals only if it has submitted to the FDA a supplemental application covering the new use, or if the manufacturer certifies that it will soon submit such a supplement, or in the unlikely event that the FDA grants an exemption from the supplement requirement. In essence, the provision offers at most a minimal acceleration of approval of submitted or soon-to-be-submitted supplemental applications. At the same time, the FDA's discretion in these matters provides yet another stick for regulators to use on drug companies.

Substantial relief on the off-label use issue came to drug manufacturers, health care professionals, and patients but not through legislation. It resulted from an August 1998 federal court decision, *Washington Legal Foundation* v. *Friedman*, which struck down on First Amendment constitutional grounds the FDA's prohibition against drug manufacturers distributing peer-reviewed medical literature.[14] The court found that whereas the FDA could properly block drug companies from distributing *their own* marketing materials to physicians if they describe non-FDA-approved uses, it is an infringement of their commercial speech rights to prevent them from handing out journal articles, textbooks, and the like that describe new uses for a drug already approved for other purposes. The federal judiciary has thereby pushed back the FDA regulatory juggernaut where Congress was unwilling to do so—and in a case brought not by a drug company, trade association, or patient group but by a nonprofit, public service organization.

After the court's ruling, the FDA moved to block the decision, arguing that the court had addressed a policy superseded by FDAMA and asking the court to declare that it need not adhere to the constitutional principles cited in the court's opinion. The agency further argued that the new law only permits a manufacturer to distribute materials about off-label uses if it has begun the process of getting supplemental FDA approval for the new use,[15] and in November 1998 the FDA effectively ignored the court's ruling and adopted regulations reimposing the restrictions, claiming that the new regulations should not be subject to the judge's injunction because they were adopted pursuant to FDAMA. (So much for the FDA's commitment to regulatory reform.) In July 1999, the federal court categorically rejected that argument and held that the new FDA regulations and the FDAMA provision under which the new regulations were adopted were unconstitutional. The court angrily dismissed the FDA's argument that its restrictions were not subject to First Amendment constitutional limitations, calling it "of course, preposterous."[16] (So much for the FDA's commitment to the

14. *Washington Legal Foundation* v. *Friedman*, 94-1306 (D.D.C., filed July 30, 1998).

15. D. E. Troy, "FDA Censorship Could Cost Lives," *Wall Street Journal*, July 23, 1999, A14.

16. Washington Legal Foundation, *Court Expands Decision Striking Down FDA Speech Restrictions* (Washington, D.C.:Washington Legal Foundation, July 20, 1999) (litigation update).

rule of law.) At the same time, the court emphasized that the agency was still free to take actions to suppress false and misleading speech and that it could still require manufacturers to attach disclaimers to all distributed materials about off-label usage in order to notify health professionals that the use was not yet FDA approved.[17]

The bill does contains some minor improvements. Section 114(a), for example, permits manufacturers to submit "health care economic information," such as data on a drug's cost-effectiveness, to hospitals and health maintenance organizations—in effect removing a restriction that should not have existed in the first place. This change will enable information to flow more freely, boosting the efficiency of cooperation among various players in the drug production-distribution pipeline and, in a modest way, help hold down health care costs. Other provisions will loosen restrictions on health claims for food products and expand the use of third parties, including academic institutions, to review medical devices. But among such small beneficial changes is one devious provision. Section 410 actually *increases* the scope of FDA regulation by expanding the agency's jurisdiction to cover activities that pertain to any potentially regulated product and that occur completely within a single state. Before this change in the law, *intrastate* research or treatment generally was not subject to federal regulations; now, for regulatory purposes, all such activities are considered to be *interstate* commerce. For the first time, the FDA will have explicit regulatory authority over small-scale research by an academic or practicing physician whose testing of an innovative drug therapy is performed wholly within a single state.

In sum, most of the supposedly significant improvements in FDAMA do little more than codify small changes that had already been made by the FDA, and none of the genuinely new modifications mandated by the legislation will significantly improve total development times, costs, or the availability of products to patients. Moreover, the agency's actions during the more than three years since FDAMA's enactment

17. Ibid.

illustrate the need for genuine and fundamental reform. Nothing has changed—at least not for the better. As discussed below, through reckless rule making and blatant disregard for the negative impacts of its actions, the FDA continues to arrogate greater control over the health care industry and to raise the bar for drug manufacturers.

Post-FDAMA, Regulatory Creep Creeps On

FDA's War on Relationships

In January 1998, just two months after the president signed FDAMA, and while the FDA's public relations apparatus was still proclaiming the agency's commitment to regulatory reform and moderation, the FDA resumed its power creep. The agency published a draft guidance document aimed at regulating "medical product promotion" among health care providers and professionals.[18] Although the proposal's stated goal is to deter pharmaceutical manufacturers from unfairly promoting their own products through health care organizations and insurers, the FDA policy exerts a chilling effect on the beneficial exchange of information among various segments of the health care industry and could eventually interfere with essential communication between health care providers and patients. Moreover, it is hopelessly vague, duplicates regulatory functions already being performed by other government agencies, and exceeds the FDA's statutory mandate.

The FDA's statutory authority encompasses a manufacturer's product labeling and advertising, primarily to deter labeling or advertising that is false or misleading. This is not unreasonable, given the FDA's mandate. The new policy, however, would extend the agency's regulatory authority to any "relationships" among health care professionals it deems promotional. Not only does this go beyond the FDA's legal

18. Food and Drug Administration, Department of Health and Human Service, "Promoting Medical Products in a Changing Healthcare Environment: Medical Product Promotion by Healthcare Organizations or Pharmacy Benefits Management Companies (PBMs)," *Federal Register* 63 (January 5, 1998): 236–39.

authority, but the wording of the proposal is so ambiguous that it could effectively shut down vital communication among health care professionals and patients. For example, the FDA argues that if any "subsidiary" of a drug manufacturer promotes a drug, the parent company bears full legal responsibility. But the agency says that "subsidiary" is "to be interpreted in its broadest sense to include any corporate relationship," no matter how remote, and that a company involved in a relationship with "an independent contractor or agent becomes responsible criminally for the failure of the person to whom he has delegated the obligation to comply with the law." (The manufacturer is responsible—that is, shares the legal blame—even if it neither approved nor had knowledge of the actions in question.) Consider the following scenario: While dispensing a prescription, a pharmacist working in a store that has a remote corporate relationship with a drug manufacturer gives a patient information about the use of an FDA-approved drug but for a purpose not yet sanctioned by the FDA. (Some 40 to 50 percent of all drugs are prescribed for such off-label uses, including 60 to 70 percent of drugs used to treat cancer and 90 percent of drugs used in pediatrics.)[19] According to the FDA's new policy, the manufacturer, the pharmacist, and possibly any middlemen could all be cited for violations of the FDA's regulations.

The FDA proposal intrudes into areas where other agencies already protect the consumer, so the FDA cannot claim to be filling a regulatory void. State attorneys general and the Federal Trade Commission set industry standards for disclosure of a manufacturer's relationships, for example. Clinical programs are regulated by state boards of medicine and pharmacy. The federal Health Care Finance Administration regulates reimbursement, discounting, self-referral, kickbacks, fraud, and abuse under rules that bind all health care organizations. These regulatory bodies are better suited to monitor relationships among health

19. David R. Henderson, *FDA Censorship Can Be Hazardous to Your Health*, Policy Brief 158 (St. Louis, Mo.: Center for the Study of American Business, September 1995).

care organizations and providers than the FDA, whose mission is (or should be) to assure the safety and efficacy of products.

Rules on Reporting Drug Side Effects

Neither FDAMA nor the FDA's ostensible self-reform has caused the agency to reconsider an arguably unnecessary proposal that illustrates how regulators' unchecked risk aversion and discretion are translated into vast expense to drug developers (and, ultimately, to patients). In 1995 the FDA proposed a new rule (that still had not been issued in final form by May 2000) that would mandate new, expanded reporting requirements on the side effects of drugs in clinical trials.[20] This regulation was the brainchild of FDA commissioner David Kessler, who directed that it be prepared despite significant opposition within the agency. Kessler was (over-) reacting to a 1994 incident with an experimental drug called fialuridine, or FIAU, which was being tested for the treatment of chronic active hepatitis. During the clinical testing sponsored by the National Institutes of Health (NIH), the drug actually worsened liver failure in dozens of patients, causing several deaths and requiring liver transplants in others. Because the side effects were similar to the usual progression of the illness, it was difficult at first to ascertain whether the drug was causing those problems. Under the new regulation, the FDA will require more frequent reporting of side effects and also require notification not only to the agency but to research institutions' institutional review boards, which are ill equipped for such an avalanche of paperwork. The regulation will reconfigure the burden of proof so that if a patient gets sick or sicker during any clinical trial, the experimental drug will be assumed to be the cause until another cause can be identified; one might say that all new drugs will be presumed guilty until conclusively proven innocent. This change in the burden

20. Food and Drug Administration, Department of Health and Human Services, "Adverse Experience Reporting Requirements for Human Drug and Licensed Biological Products," *Federal Register* 59 (October 27, 1994): 54046–64.

of proof ignores the fact that often in clinical trials it is not the medication being tested that causes injury to the patient but some other factor—although that alternative etiology is often not readily provable. The FDA's new policy also ignores two analyses of the FIAU incident, one by the NIH and the other by the prestigious Institute of Medicine, neither of which found any deficiency in the existing system for reporting side effects.[21] The proposed change in the reporting of side effects and the new, lower regulatory threshold for stopping a clinical trial will make the entire drug development process even more risk averse, slower, and more expensive.

Medical researchers at the Johns Hopkins University Center for Clinical Trials, led by Dr. Curtis L. Meinert, carefully compared two clinical trials, one performed with reporting according to the old requirements and one under the proposed rules. They concluded that the FDA's proposed changes would increase the cost per patient and the paperwork generated per patient to an extraordinary extent: On a per patient basis, the costs increased from $151 to $9,407—a whopping 62-fold increase; and the paperwork increased from 135 to 8,500 pages—a 63-fold increase![22] The researchers concluded that the hugely increased costs and complexity of clinical trials would not be accompanied by commensurate advantages to patients. In their submitted comments on the proposed regulation, the Dupont-Merck Pharmaceutical Company estimated that the reporting burden would double for each prospective drug in development, and Amgen, Inc., described the practical difficulties of estimating the expected incidences of death and serious adverse events that arise, not from the drug, but from underlying disease or concomitant medications.[23] Consider, for example, that in a terminal

21. Frederick J. Manning and Morton Swartz, eds., *Review of the Fialuridine (FIAU) Trials* (Washington D.C.: National Academy Press, 1995).

22. Curtis L. Meinert, "An Open Letter to the FDA Regarding Changes in Reporting Procedures for Drugs and Biologics Proposed in the Wake of the FIAU Tragedy," *Controlled Clinical Trials* 17 (1996): 273–84.

23. Official docket for public comments on, "Adverse Experience Reporting Requirements for Human Drug and Licensed Biological Products," *Federal Register* 59 (October 27, 1994): 54046–64, Food and Drug Administration, Rockville, Maryland, 20856.

cancer patient with multiple organ failure, an episode of lightheaded-ness, cardiac arrhythmia, or an abnormal laboratory finding could be due to the test drug, another drug the patient is taking, the metabolic derangements of the underlying disease itself, or a new, unrelated ill-ness.

Compulsory Testing of Drugs on Children

In November 1998 the FDA announced that drug companies would thenceforth be required to test on children the medicines they sell for adults and to put the pediatric dosages on the label.[24] That might sound benign, or even desirable, but these new requirements ignore the real-ities of drug testing and impose quantitatively and qualitatively new burdens on drug developers. The new requirement may actually be detrimental to children and could delay the availability of new drugs if the FDA withholds approval for adult uses while the required data from pediatric studies are being collected. The regulation is a rigid, central-ized governmental solution to a nonproblem, according to many pedi-atricians. The FDA itself concedes that, using data obtained solely from adult clinical trials, physicians commonly and safely prescribe pain relievers, asthma drugs, antihistamines, antibiotics, and other therapeu-tics many millions of times annually for children. Even if additional testing of drugs in children were needed, there are more inventive and effective (and market-oriented) ways to accomplish it than the FDA's heavy-handed approach. For example, the FDA could simply require a prominent label or logo on drug preparations whose safety and efficacy have not yet been determined in children, or the agency could publish a list of such drugs annually. This would make parents and physicians

24. Food and Drug Administration, Department of Health and Human Services, "Regulations Requiring Manufacturers to Assess the Safety and Effectiveness of New Drugs and Biological Products in Pediatric Patients; Final Rule, FDA," *Federal Register* 63 (December 2, 1998): 66632–72.

aware that such information is not available, and they, in turn, could exert moral and economic pressure on drug companies to obtain it. Or conversely, the FDA could permit a distinguishing label or logo to identify those products that had been tested in children. (Consider that it is in drug companies' interests both to avoid harming patients and to expand the population that will purchase and benefit from their products.)

The regulation makes no allowance for the fact that creating a dosage form appropriate for children is often especially challenging. The product has to taste good enough that children will actually take it, a requirement that might necessitate clinical studies of a new pediatric formulation. Also children's medications are often in a chewable or syrup form, but such new formulations can raise questions about special storage requirements and adequate shelf life. Finally, clinical trials are difficult to perform with children. For ethical reasons, the initial (phase I) testing is done in children who are ill, not in healthy volunteers. Study participants may be scarce because a disease is rare in children, because the population is geographically diverse, or because parents are reluctant to enroll their sick children in an experiment. For the purposes of drug testing, the designation "children" is by no means a homogenous category. The term implies several groups that are physiologically and metabolically distinct: newborns, infants, preschoolers, primary schoolers, and teens. Moreover, children may pass through two or more age groups during the course of a multiyear clinical study, confounding statistical analysis.

Finally, the regulation appears to go beyond the FDA's traditional responsibility to certify drugs and assure that sponsor-generated data demonstrate safety and efficacy before a product is marketed. The FDA appears to be expropriating the prerogative of sponsors to make strategic decisions about whether and when to pursue certain labeling indications for their drugs. This is yet another example of the FDA continuing to push the regulatory envelope.

It is clear from the FDA's recent regulations and regulatory interpretations that the agency's pretense of a commitment to regulatory reform—a political necessity with a Republican-controlled Congress since 1995—has not translated into genuine benefits to industrial innovators or to patients. The agency has continued to propose and implement rules and policies that add further costs and time to the development of new drugs, with little or no additional consumer protection. If there is ever to be true reform, it will have to come from outside the FDA. The current regulatory system, cobbled together over more than six decades, is a confusing, draconian mosaic of mandates, requirements, interpretations, and precedents under a centralized government monopoly whose power and scope have increased unremittingly. Along the way, Congress's original concept of how drug development should be regulated has been distorted, but the public—and Congress, for that matter—has shown little desire for genuine reform. Still, the tides of public policy, like those of fashion, are fickle, and when the tides of public opinion and congressional sentiment eventually flow back toward a desire to make drug regulation more efficient (stimulated, in all likelihood, by sticker shock over constantly increasing prices), it will be useful to have available a comprehensive regulatory model that maintains high product standards, and reduces the costs and delays in drug development. Such a model is described in part 2.

PART 2

A MODEL FOR
REFORM OF THE
FOOD AND DRUG
ADMINISTRATION

5

A Spectrum of Possibilities

The FDA's apparent indifference to the interests of both consumers and industry would not have been possible were it not for the agency's regulatory monopoly over food, drug, and medical device regulation and the absence of effective oversight by Congress. There is nothing sacrosanct about government monopolies performing premarket regulation, however; a wide range of institutional models for drug regulation exists. At the opposite pole from a government monopoly is laissez-faire, a self-regulating system in which government has no role at all and all decisions about testing and marketing are made unilaterally by drug manufacturers. Between the two extremes, other institutional alternatives offer various configurations of government oversight and nongovernment mechanisms for the regulation and monitoring of the nation's supply of new drugs. These alternative organizational arrangements involve varying degrees of privatization and FDA control of the certification process.

Recent history provides evidence of the failures of the two extremes of monopoly and laissez-faire to serve the public interest; abuse of power is too easy in both. Government monopolies foster abuses by bureaucrats; laissez-faire creates similar temptations for companies, with obvious risk to the public. Proponents of laissez-faire maintain that, in the absence of government oversight, companies would be induced to protect the integrity of their products by goodwill, a desire to preserve their reputations, and the fear of civil litigation (and even possible criminal prosecution). But, inevitably, some drug manufacturers would take dangerous shortcuts in manufacturing, testing, or surveillance; and, although an acceptable level of safety might be achieved much of the time, where issues of health and safety are concerned even rare failures would lead to reregulation by government. The public reaction to isolated incidents of poisonings that led to the Biologics Act of 1902 and the Federal Food, Drug and Cosmetic Act of 1938 (see chapter 1) illustrates the infeasibility of a laissez-faire system. Even with the existing FDA monopoly and stringency of regulation, occasional high-profile mishaps stimulate ever-greater regulatory burdens.

If the extremes are unworkable, what other models are available? One possible arrangement would simply remove the FDA's veto power over new products, creating a kind of laissez-faire system but with an optional FDA review offering a Good Housekeeping–like seal of approval. Another option would be a *private* monopoly organization to review and certify new products under the FDA's oversight. Still another would have drug manufacturers contract with private entities to assume many of the functions currently performed by the FDA, with private firms competing, under FDA oversight, to supply evaluation and certification services.[1]

To be accepted by American consumers, any system needs to incorporate a more-or-less independent review of product safety and probably of effectiveness as well. According to the 1996 analysis by the Progress & Freedom Foundation of such possible arrangements for regulation (which I coauthored), the most efficient and workable model for reform is the last of those enumerated above—a system that has competing private bodies certifying drugs under government oversight.[2] This ar-

1. Robert D. Tollison, "Institutional Alternatives for the Regulation of Drugs and Medical Devices," in Ralph A. Epstein et al., *Advancing Medical Innovation: Health, Safety, and the Role of Government in the 21st Century* (Washington, D.C.: Progress & Freedom Foundation, 1996), pp. 17–37.
2. Ibid.

rangement would have nongovernmental entities performing the primary oversight of clinical testing and the initial assessment of whether the criteria for safety and efficacy have been met, and the FDA would confer the final sign-off on marketing approval. These entities, called drug certifying bodies, or DCBs, would assume many of the evaluative and consultative functions now performed by the FDA during product testing and review; the agency would be transformed from a *certifier of products* into a *certifier of certifiers*.[3]

In many respects, this approach resembles the current European system for the oversight of medical devices and the U.S. nationally recognized testing laboratories (NRTLs), which set standards for and certify thousands of categories of products and commodities (*vide infra*). This system would yield more rapid approval of beneficial new drugs, while maintaining the current legal standards of safety and efficacy. Moreover, it would allow governmental drug review bodies in certain other countries, such as the United Kingdom, to act as certifying bodies in the United States. That is to say, approval of a new drug by the U.K.'s regulatory authority would be tantamount to a recommendation for approval by a U.S.-based DCB. This additional level of competition would constitute a variant of reciprocal approvals among various nations' regulatory authorities and would provide a further stimulus to new products entering the U.S. market.

Medical Device Regulation: Lessons for Drug Regulation

The regulation of medical devices in the European Union relies heavily on various sets of product standards. Manufacturing and quality control standards are strict, and record-keeping and reporting requirements, rigorous. Should a problem develop, manufacturers must provide all available documentation and cooperate fully with regulatory authorities. Normally, however, government involvement is minimal. The vast

3. DCBs were first described in Epstein et al., *Advancing Medical Innovation*.

majority of products require no clinical trials or external premarket approval, and manufacturers are allowed a great deal of flexibility in how they meet the standards. For low-risk devices, manufacturers themselves are allowed to certify that their products meet the necessary standards (self-certification). For higher-risk products (such as cardiac pacemakers and X-ray machines) manufacturers must seek certification from third parties, so-called notified bodies,[4] which test products, inspect manufacturing systems, and ultimately certify that European Union (EU) standards have been met. Following this certification, the product can be marketed. In other words, approval of a product by a notified body is tantamount to government approval. The notified bodies themselves are subject to oversight by national governments with respect to their operations as certifiers. In addition, as in the United States, postmarketing reporting to national authorities of adverse incidents is required. Such incidents must be reported by manufacturers and users, and, in consultation with national government authorities, the manufacturer must decide how to manage the risk. These decisions can range from changing the indications or use of the product to removing it from the market.

The European experience demonstrates the viability of a graduated regulatory system that includes government-established standards and a combination of manufacturers' self-certification and independent third-party certification. This has important implications for regulation in the United States, where an analogous approach could produce not only a marked improvement over the current system for the oversight of medical devices but also serve as a model for drug regulation. Under pressure to improve its performance, the FDA has already completed a pilot program (which ended in November 1998) that allowed third-party review of certain medical devices—those not permanently implantable, not life sustaining or life supporting, and not requiring clinical data for clearance. On the termination of the pilot program, under

4. Ralph A. Epstein, "Medical Devices," in Epstein et al., *Advancing Medical Innovation*, pp. 59–77.

a new "third-party review program" established under FDAMA, the FDA began to permit the review of specified medical devices by certain nongovernmental "accredited persons."[5] The number of products eligible for this outside review was increased by FDAMA, but even with these modifications the U.S. system falls far short of the breadth and advantages of the European model.

It is noteworthy that both the theory and practice of the FDA's own third-party review for medical devices are consistent with the proposal in this volume to apply nongovernmental, expert review to drugs:

> The purpose of this program is to implement section 523 of the [FDA Modernization Act of 1997] by accrediting third parties (Accredited Persons) to conduct the initial review of 510(k)s [applications reviewed by the FDA, or an accredited person, for a determination that a new device is substantially equivalent to a predicate device, in which case the new device is in the same class and may be introduced to the market subject to the same regulatory controls as its predicate device] for selected low-to-moderate risk devices. The Third Party Review Pilot Program now under way will terminate on November 21, 1998, which is when FDA will begin accepting reviews and recommendations from trained Accredited Persons.
>
> The Accredited Persons program will enable FDA to target its scientific review resources at higher-risk devices, while maintaining a high degree of confidence in the review process by using Accredited Persons to assess low-to-moderate risk devices and at the same time provide manufacturers of eligible devices an alternative review process that may yield more rapid 510(k) decisions. In accordance with the requirements of section 523 and based on experience with the Third Party Review Pilot Program, the Accredited Person Review Program includes a number of features designed to maintain a high level of quality in 510(k)s reviewed by Accredited Persons and to minimize risks to the public. These include: . . . Personnel qualifications for Accredited Persons equivalent to the level within CDRH's [Center for Devices and Radiological Health] Of-

---

5. See, for example, the lists of eligible devices and accredited persons at www.fda.gov/cdrh/dsma/3rdpty.html, accessed on the FDA's web site, October 28, 1999.

fice of Device Evaluation; criteria to prevent potential conflicts of interest for Accredited Persons that might affect the review process; FDA oversight of Accredited Person reviews/recommendations and FDA's continued responsibility for the issuance of 510(k) decisions; provisions for FDA to make onsite visits on a periodic basis to each Accredited Person to audit performance and for inspection of records, correspondence, and other materials relating to Accredited Person review; FDA monitoring and evaluation of the program to ensure that Accredited Persons are substantially in compliance with the requirements of section 523 of the act and do not pose a threat to public health; continued applicability of all other regulatory controls (e.g., medical device reporting of post-marketing adverse events) applicable to devices included in the program; prohibition against forum shopping by subcommittees of 510(k)s; and use of review guidance and/or recognized standards to ensure accurate and timely review by Accredited Persons. The purpose of a review by an Accredited Person is to evaluate a manufacturer's 510(k), document the review, and make a recommendation to FDA concerning the substantial equivalence of the device or initial classification under 513(f)(1). FDA will provide information on procedures and criteria that it uses for 510(k) reviews in general guidance and in a training program to be made available by FDA before commencement of the program.[6]

This third-party review by accredited persons is a welcome—albeit conservative—step toward privatization of the oversight of medical devices, and the model proposed in this volume is its logical extension to the regulation of drugs.

The Nationally Recognized Testing
Laboratories Model

In the United States, there is already a long-standing and highly successful private-sector certification system for various consumer and industrial products that has much in common with the European system

6. Center for Devices and Radiological Health, Food and Drug Administration, *Guidance for Staff, Industry, and Third Parties: Implementation of Third Party Programs under the FDA Modernization Act of 1997* (Washington, D.C.:Food and Drug Administration, October 30, 1998).

for medical device oversight. The prototype of this system of national recognized testing laboratories (NRTLs) is Underwriters Laboratories (UL), a large, not-for-profit organization that tests and certifies products, many of which present inherent potential hazards to life and property.[7] It certifies more than 16,500 types of products, including electrical appliances and equipment, automotive and mechanical products, fire-resistant building materials, and bullet-resistant glass. Using more than 650 discrete standards, or guidelines, the UL certification offers assurance of safety but not of effectiveness (except in a few special cases where the two factors are inextricably linked, such as fire extinguishers and smoke detectors). Each standard is a detailed specification for a single product class. New standards are written as market demand requires them. As the demand for UL certification of a certain product class arises, the organization prepares a draft of suggested testing procedures and criteria that products must meet in order to receive certification. This information is distributed for comment to interested bodies, such as groups of manufacturers, insurers, and consumers, before a "proposed standard" is drafted. This proposed standard then undergoes another round of review and deliberation and culminates in a perfected "published standard," which is made available to manufacturers. A fee is charged for the UL's services, based on the complexity and cost of testing products in a given category. UL and its competitors—other NRTLs—are certified and regulated by the Occupational Safety and Health Administration (OSHA), an agency of the U.S. Department of Labor.[8]

Not all NRTLs are standard-setting bodies. Many use UL's standards directly and offer to manufacturers some compensating differential in cost or ancillary services to attract business. Some set their own standards

7. www.ul.com/, accessed November 19, 1999.

8. Occupational Safety and Health Administration (OSHA), Department of Labor, "Definition of Nationally Recognized Testing Laboratory; Determination of Eligible Testing Organizations" (29 CFR, Parts 1907 and 1910), *Federal Register* 53 (April 12, 1988): 12102–25; *Federal Register* 53 (May 11, 1988): 16838; as amended at *Federal Register* 54 (June 7, 1989): 24333; *Federal Register* 61 (February 13, 1996): 5507.

and testing protocols, independent of the actions of the UL, although competing standards do not vary greatly. Typically, UL's direct competitors are smaller, newer, and for-profit enterprises. The UL's not-for-profit status is the result of its curious history and inception. Since its beginning, the UL's stated mission has been "testing for public safety,"[9] and although UL receives fees to defray the costs of testing and overhead, its activities have always been defined as a public service. As a testing and certifying organization, UL does not underwrite any risk of the products it certifies. Nor are its liability concerns excessive; as an independent third party UL is not jointly liable for any defects in the product's performance in situ, and UL certification does not legally connect the organization to any negligence by the manufacturer.

NRTLs are completely private and independent, and manufacturers contract with them for certification services on a wholly voluntary basis. NRTLs hold no monopoly on safety certification, and their approvals are not equivalent to government approval. However, many retailers are reluctant to carry products lacking UL (or equivalent) approval, and, occasionally, insurers deny liability coverage for products without it. Manufacturers, insurers, and the NRTLs all have incentives to maintain high standards both for consumer products and for the companies that make them.

The NRTL Model Applied to Drug Approval

The successes of NRTL certification and the European system for regulating medical devices suggest the applicability of a government-supervised private certification system to the oversight of drugs, as does the third-party review of certain medical devices in the United States (*vide supra*).[10] To be sure, more is involved in the development and review of new drugs (and some medical devices) than simply testing a batch of products according to manufacturing or performance stan-

---

9. Ibid.
10. Robert D. Tollison, "Speeding Drug Approvals, Safely Privately," *Consumers Research* (January 1998): 14–16.

dards; that is, meeting production standards is not sufficient. In most instances, at the beginning of clinical trials of drugs there is genuine uncertainty about their ultimate outcome. For example, the product might prove to have an unfavorable benefit/risk profile; it might perform poorly when compared with alternative therapies, or it might simply not be effective. (Only about 20 percent of drugs that enter clinical trials are ultimately approved for marketing.)[11] Such conceptual differences between drugs and other products notwithstanding, given the legal right to do so it is conceivable that some NRTLs and other organizations could expand their capabilities to undertake drug testing. They would need to acquire experts who could evaluate data from laboratory, preclinical (animal), and clinical studies and who could perform the appropriate audits to assure the accuracy and fidelity of the data, but this is certainly feasible.

A model for the evaluation of clinical data by an independent organization already exists. In a two-year (1992–1994) pilot program undertaken at the urging of the Bush administration's Council on Competitiveness, the FDA contracted out reviews of NDA supplements and compared the results of these evaluations to in-house analyses.[12] The contractor was the Mitre Corporation (now Mitre-Tek), a nonprofit technical consulting company. In all five supplements reviewed by Mitre, the recommendations were completely congruent with the FDA's own evaluations. Moreover, the time required for the reviews was two to four months, and the cost ranged from $20,000 to $70,000 — fast and cheap compared to federal regulators.

As well as providing a model, this pilot program serves as a reminder that the FDA has at one time or another delegated virtually every part of its various review and evaluation functions (except the final sign-off of marketing approval) to outside expert advisors, consultants, or other entities. It also is a reminder that the delegation generally has been piecemeal, disorganized, and short lived, as well as wildly unpopular

11. Anon., *New Drug Approvals* (Washington D.C.: Pharmaceutical Research and Manufacturers Association, January 1998), p. 18.

12. Testimony of Pamela Walker, Mitre-Tek Systems, before the Committee on Labor and Human Resources of the U.S. Senate, February 21, 1996.

within the agency. The FDA has completely ignored the success of the Mitre reviews, and because such programs have not been encouraged by the Clinton White House, there has been no follow-up.

A central and essential element of the EU and NRTL oversight models is competition for clients—that is, manufacturers who need product certification. Experience has shown repeatedly that such competition keeps costs down without compromising quality. For example, an analysis of trends in the cost of wireless telephone service in northern California concluded that "the price break that's drawing . . . thousands of casual users to mobile phones resulted from newly vigorous competition in the [San Francisco] Bay Area. Three wireless carriers have moved into the market in the past two years, driving down prices some 30 percent in the past year alone."[13] In their separate spheres, the NRTLs and the EU's notified bodies similarly compete for clients among manufacturers, just as the EMEA and European national regulatory agencies compete against one another.

NRTLs and the accredited third parties who participate in medical device regulation as specified in FDAMA may be for profit or nonprofit; in the EU the notified bodies involved in medical device oversight are all commercial, profit-making organizations.

Were it to be implemented, the proposal made here would spark healthy competition. There would be potent incentives to form DCBs and high demand for services. The primary incentive to create a DCB would, of course, be the desire to share in the more than $25 billion annually spent on drug research and development in the United States. Several kinds of existing organizations could serve as the nidus for DCBs. In addition to the NRTLs like Underwriters Laboratories and private consulting firms like Mitre-Tek, there are medical schools and other university-based centers like the Johns Hopkins Center for the Study of Clinical Trials. There are also clinical research organizations (CROs), which currently perform clinical studies under contract to

13. Jon Healey, "Cell Phone Market Explodes," *San Jose Mercury News*, January 5, 1999, A1.

drug companies. (Because of conflict-of-interest considerations, however, a single entity would be prohibited from both performing studies and evaluating them.) Many of these organizations already have experts in many of the disciplines required by DCBs: pharmaceutical toxicology, pharmaceutical formulations, biopharmaceutics, medical subspecialties, molecular biology, drug study design, clinical monitoring of therapeutics and quality assurance, chemistry, statistics, manufacturing, and the legal aspects of regulation. These kinds of organizations, plus the FDA, National Institutes of Health, Centers for Disease Control and Prevention, and other government agencies, constitute a large pool of potential scientific and medical experts, entrepreneurs, and administrators who could populate DCBs. Similar to the periods of rapid growth of biotech companies in the 1970s and 1980s and of HMOs in the 1980s and 1990s, the attraction of lucrative businesses will be an irresistible lure.

Although hypothetically a "race to the bottom" could occur if some DCBs attempted to attract clients by doing quick-and-dirty reviews and granting approvals prematurely, several factors militate against that possibility. First, the desire to maintain a reputation as a competent testing organization is a potent market incentive and exerts a strong influence on the behavior of private certification laboratories. Second, the FDA's certification authority over the DCBs, as well as the veto power it will retain over their recommendations, should act as a strong deterrent. Third, there is the threat of litigation for negligence, and even criminal prosecution, should harm result from an inadequately or negligently evaluated product. Finally, scenarios that postulate conspiracies between greedy and unscrupulous drug developers and regulators belie the experience of NRTLs in the United States and notified bodies in Europe.

6

A Proposal for
Regulatory Reform

In this section, fundamental changes to the existing U.S. drug approval system are proposed, some of whose basic elements first emerged from the study of drug regulation by the Progress & Freedom Foundation[1] referred to in previous chapters. These changes would create a system that is more efficient and more focused on the needs of public health. Their implementation would require congressional amendment of existing statutes—not an easy task in the best of circumstances—but the positive impacts would be considerable. The overall time and cost required to bring safe and effective new products to market would be reduced; a more appropriate balance between regulation and innovation would be restored; and competition would be stimulated. Most important, the overall effect of these reforms would be to get a greater number of drugs to patients more expeditiously and at lower cost.

---

1. Ralph A. Epstein et al., *Advancing Medical Innovation: Health, Safety, and the Role of Government in the 21st Century* (Washington, D.C.: Progress & Freedom Foundation, 1996).

The Current System of Drug
Development and Regulation

The proposed system does not dismantle the processes and institutions now in place that perform the evaluation of new drugs. Rather, it shifts some roles and responsibilities from government to private entities, builds in a government-based appeals process to adjudicate disagreements, and takes some logical steps toward full reciprocity with certain foreign regulatory agencies. To understand the importance of the changes, some familiarity with the details — and shortcomings — of the present system is necessary.

The initial "discovery" of a new drug in the laboratory, as well as subsequent development and testing, is performed not by the FDA but by a sponsor, usually a private pharmaceutical company. In a small percentage of cases a federal agency, university, hospital, or research institution might undertake product discovery, obtain a patent, and start development, but seldom do such entities have the resources and specialized skills to take a drug through the full development process to marketing approval.

Development of a new drug generally begins with in vitro screening for desired chemical or biological activity, followed by testing in laboratory animals to determine therapeutic activity and possible toxicities (see figure 7). These *preclinical* investigations generate preliminary knowledge about the pharmacological and toxicological properties of the agent and also help to predict possible uses for it and the initial dose range for humans in clinical trials. Many compounds are eliminated from further development at this stage. If animal studies suggest that a compound may be therapeutically promising, the sponsor moves on to clinical testing — that is, administration of the drug to human subjects. At this point the first of two basic applications to the FDA must be made. Before introducing the drug for the first time into humans (or into certain new subpopulations, such as children or pregnant women), the sponsor must apply for approval of an Investigational New Drug, or IND, filing. The agency has thirty days to review the submission and

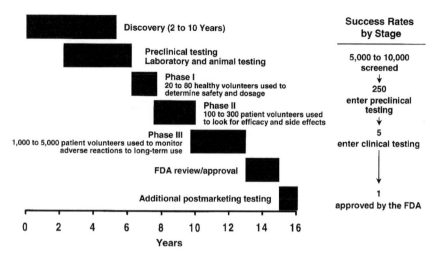

Figure 7. Stages and Success Rates of the Clinical Testing of Drugs.
Source: Joseph A. DiMasi, "Success Rates for New Drugs Entering Clinical Testing in the United States," *Clinical Pharmacology and Therapeutics* 58 (1995): 1–14.

evaluate whether risk/benefit considerations support the proposed re-search in human subjects. If the FDA does not formally object by the end of that period, the sponsor may begin clinical testing.

Although drug development, in practice, is a continuum of research (see figure 7), the process of *clinical testing*—the most resource-inten-sive phase of drug development (see figure 8)—can be thought of as consisting of several discrete phases. Phase I is often the initial admin-istration of a drug to human subjects (as few as a dozen subjects, usually healthy volunteers). Phase II studies are generally the first exposure of the target patient population to the drug, and they commonly involve from a few dozen to a few hundred patients. By the time phase II is completed, the data usually indicate whether the drug offers sufficient promise to warrant larger-scale (expanded phase II or phase III) clinical trials. Phase III trials are carried out when there is a significant expec-tation the product ultimately will be approved by the FDA and mar-keted. These expanded trials attempt to ascertain (1) the drug's effec-tiveness in a larger number and broader spectrum of patients and, often,

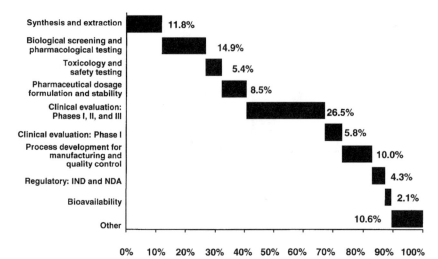

Figure 8. Where the Drug Research and Development (R&D) Dollar Goes.
Source: Pharmaceutical Research and Manufacturers of America, *1999 Industry Profile* (Washington, D.C.: PhRMA, 1999), p. 22. *Note:* Totals may not add exactly due to rounding. R&D functions are not exactly sequential in practice.

a wider range of disease conditions, or "indications"; (2) the kinds and frequency of side effects in a larger and more heterogenous population; (3) the potential for long-term use; (4) interactions with other drugs; and (5) other information useful for drug labeling. These phase III trials are generally the longest and most costly component of clinical trials, often involving from several hundred to many thousands of patients and costing tens of millions, or even hundreds of millions, of dollars.[2] (One cardiovascular drug failed in a multicenter phase III clinical trial after the expenditure of a quarter-billion dollars.)[3] Only about one out of three of the drugs that begins clinical testing survives to enter phase III,

2. Pharmaceutical Research and Manufacturers of America, *Pharmaceutical Industry 1999* (Washington, D.C.: Pharmaceutical Research and Manufacturers of America), p. 22.
3. Henry I. Miller and William M. Wardell, "Therapeutic Drugs and Biologics," in Epstein et al., *Advancing Medical Innovation*, p. 57.

and only about one out of five drugs that enters clinical testing ultimately is approved for marketing.[4]

Studies described as phase I may have to be done or repeated after phase II or even phase III has begun. For example, after advanced clinical testing in adults, the sponsor might decide to seek a pediatric indication, which could necessitate new phase I and II studies in children, especially if the formulation is significantly changed. Often, many different types of studies with a drug candidate are done simultaneously—different stages of testing in various patient populations for multiple indications—with the studies proceeding at different rates. Still, the three phases represent a logical, if somewhat idealized, progression of size and complexity

When clinical testing has been completed and the data analyzed, if the drug sponsor is satisfied that the drug's safety and effectiveness for a given indication have been demonstrated, it seeks approval to market the drug by submitting to the FDA a New Drug Application, or NDA (or the similar Biologics Licensing Application, BLA, in the case of a biological drug). The NDA submission includes a description of the drug's composition; the methods, facilities, and controls for the manufacturing, processing, and packaging of the drug; samples of the drug and its components; and a draft version of the proposed labeling. It also includes a complete and detailed report of all investigations and statistical analyses performed during testing. The NDA is hundreds of thousands of pages long. (Television news producers like to show footage of the thousands of volumes being unloaded from a tractor-trailer at FDA headquarters.) NDAs are reviewed at the FDA's Center for Drug Evaluation and Research (CDER), BLAs at the Center for Biologics Evaluation and Research (CBER). The reviews are performed by teams consisting of physicians, pharmacologists, chemists, statisticians, and other specialists. By statute, the FDA is required to approve or

4. Pharmaceutical Research and Manufacturers Association, *New Drug Approvals* (Washington, D.C.: Pharmaceutical Research and Manufacturers Association, January 1998), p. 18.

disapprove an NDA within 180 days, although this deadline is rarely met. The 180-day period can be extended by "agreement" between the sponsor and the FDA. Most NDA submissions (at present 85 percent) ultimately are approved by the FDA.[5] Frequently, however, final approval comes only after considerable time and negotiation and additional submission of data. Also, the FDA may narrow the sponsor's initial request by approving the drug for fewer indications and smaller patient populations than requested by the sponsor. If a drug is not approved, there is no appeals process in place.

The effects of regulatory policies and decisions on even the early phases of drug development are important determinants of the overall time and costs of drug development. There are high attrition rates—that is, failures—of drug candidates during the early stages when little is known about them, so at any given time there are many more products under investigation at the less advanced phases. Even during the relatively brief stage of development that encompasses only IND approval and phase I clinical trials (see figure 7), the FDA can significantly impede or disrupt development. Uncertainty at this stage about whether regulators will object to the commencement of studies, request more data, or demand changes in the clinical protocol is highly disruptive and has caused many U.S. companies to shift to more predictable and favorable locations abroad for initial human testing. (The United Kingdom, for example, does not require government approval for phase I testing.) Uncertainty and confusion are common in interacting with the FDA, as Tufts University physician and researcher Louis Lasagna made clear in his study, "Improving the Drug Development Process: Needed Reforms."[6] "On almost any aspect of drug regulation that one chooses to examine, there is usually an extraordinarily wide variation in philosophy and operational procedures from division to division and

5. Joseph A. DiMasi, "Success Rates for New Drugs Entering Clinical Testing in the United States," *Clinical Pharmacology and Therapeutics* 358 (1995): 1–14.

6. Louis Lasagna, "Improving the Drug Development Process: Needed Reforms," *Drug Information Journal* 29 (1995): 415–24.

even from reviewer to reviewer," Lasagna wrote. After conducting extensive dialogues with three "experienced, top management leaders at FDA" as part of the study, Lasagna made this observation:

> One unnerving statement concerned the procedure in the Anti-inflammatory [Drugs] Division, where the Consumer Safety Officer (CSO) decided whether to grant a pre-IND meeting on the basis of "novelty of drug, sponsor's experience, and completeness of request." Since CSOs are generally not paid very well and are unlikely to be scientifically knowledgeable, they may be well suited to the general tasks of a CSO (namely, organizing meetings, keeping minutes, and other "administrative assistant" functions), but hardly seem optimally qualified to refuse a sponsor's request for a pre-IND meeting.[7]

An important corollary of Lasagna's observations applies throughout the agency. The arbitrariness and wide variation that are commonplace among FDA divisions and reviewers, coupled with the bureaucratic aversion to type 1 errors (in risk assessment parlance, those that permit a hazardous product to be marketed) cause a kind of regulators' race to the bottom. No one wants to be seen as too aggressive or too client-friendly in granting approval of clinical trials or marketing, lest he be perceived as type 1 error–prone; thus, conservatism and risk aversion become the order of the day. This underscores the importance of reforms that will promote greater consistency, efficiency, and cost reductions in the earlier phases of the drug development process. Reforms that encourage less costly, more expeditious, and unencumbered early testing could facilitate early decisions to drop compounds that will ultimately fail (that is to say, the majority) and make it possible to focus resources on the few that will succeed.

7. Ibid.

A Better Way to Regulate Drugs

The regulatory system proposed here maintains existing or equivalent standards for—and assures consumers about—product purity, potency, and quality. It retains the legal requirements for premarketing demonstration of safety and effectiveness, the FDA's final sign-off authority for product marketing, and the agency's critical involvement with overarching safety issues. However, it relies heavily on nongovernmental drug certifying bodies (DCBs) for oversight of the IND process, initial review of the NDA, and recommendation for approval. The FDA becomes, in essence, a *certifier of certifiers*, rather than a *certifier of products*. The central aspects of the proposal are these:

- The transfer of much of the day-to-day responsibility for oversight of clinical trials and review of NDAs to nongovernmental experts in DCBs

- The financing of the DCBs' oversight by user fees, via contractual arrangements between sponsors (manufacturers) and DCBs

- Competition among the DCBs for drug sponsor "clients"

- Competition also between DCBs and certain foreign regulatory agencies certified (by the FDA) to submit an approved registration package directly to the FDA and, thereby, to act as the equivalent of a U.S. DCB

No aspect of this proposal is completely new or untested; its value and innovation lie in the integration of various elements. By both offering drug sponsors the freedom to choose among certifying bodies and maintaining high standards, the proposed system will drastically change the paradigm of incentives and disincentives, risks and rewards, for those who participate in the process of drug development and its regulation. For the first time, the system will be gamed to favor policies and decisions that will make more products available more rapidly to patients.

This is how the drug development and approval process will work under the new system. The drug sponsor will hire an FDA-certified DCB that will work closely with the drug sponsor from the point in the discovery process when a product shows promise, and continue through preclinical testing and clinical trials. The DCB will issue an IND when preclinical studies indicate that risk-benefit considerations make it appropriate for clinical trials to begin. Once the research institution's institutional review board (IRB) has affirmed the decision to proceed and begin trials, the DCB will monitor the process as the product makes its way through the various phases of clinical testing. At the sponsor's request, the DCB will offer advice about the prerequisites for NDA approval and about what testing may be necessary and sufficient to demonstrate safety and efficacy, just as the FDA does currently. However, there can be no guarantee of eventual marketing approval, explicit or implicit.

If and when the clinical trials are completed to the satisfaction of the sponsor, the sponsor will seek marketing approval by submitting an NDA to the DCB for review. Once the DCB is satisfied that the product meets all FDA requirements, including the basic criteria of safety and efficacy, the DCB will send the application to the FDA with a recommendation for final approval. The DCB's recommendation will contain a detailed summary of the evidence that supports a positive recommendation. The submission will be similar to the summary basis of approval (SBA) that is currently issued by the FDA after the approval of an NDA, but it will include significantly more detail and documentation. If the FDA turns down the recommendation of the DCB, an appeals process (described below) will be available to the sponsor.

This system is designed to track the current one closely, with the exception that DCB's experts initially substitute for the FDA's, and an appeals process is included. The roles the FDA performs less efficiently and too zealously will be assumed by organizations that possess equal or greater expertise, and competition (among DCBs) will bring about a more cooperative effort by sponsor and overseer to develop useful and safe therapies and get them to the market more rapidly and cost-effectively. DCBs will have incentives to be simultaneously cooperative, careful, and conscientious. Furthermore, the devolution of responsibilities will permit the FDA to maintain and concentrate on its purview over the collection and interpretation of safety information related to drug development. Enhanced effectiveness and efficiency will suffuse the entire process.

Safety Oversight during the IND

This plan for reform retains substantial assurance of product safety. The FDA will continue to administer the present national system of pharmacovigilance—that is, the reporting of adverse drug experiences, or ADEs. The current requirements and schedules for submitting periodic and expedited safety reports will be maintained, at least for the time being. The sponsor will submit reports to the DCB, which will transmit reportable ADEs to the FDA. FDA announcements regarding safety, including any alerts based on data received by the FDA from domestic and international sources, will be made both to the DCB and to the sponsor. In this way, the DCB will have primary responsibility for oversight of the sponsor's handling of safety issues within the IND, whereas the FDA will maintain a broad purview. The FDA's role also will ensure that the agency has the information necessary for compliance with international agreements on the reporting and sharing of safety data. Although the agency will not normally be involved in individual IND programs, when there is a specific safety (or efficacy) issue that cannot be handled through the routine oversight by a competent DCB, the FDA will participate in resolving the issue. For example, the FDA and the Centers for Disease Control (CDC) would likely be involved in the selection of viral strains that should be included in each new formulation of influenza vaccine; and the FDA would be involved in overarching policy issues such as the safety of malignant cell lines used as a source of drugs or the kinds of live viral vectors that are appropriately used for human gene therapy.

In sum, the DCB will routinely oversee the day-to-day safety aspects of an individual IND, but the FDA will retain responsibility for national oversight of safety matters, particularly those that involve information outside the purview of an individual drug sponsor or DCB. The agency will focus more resources on updating approval criteria for various therapeutic categories and indications and, as technologies and therapies evolve, will participate actively in public forums along with DCBs and drug sponsors. Ongoing interactions among the FDA, sponsors, and DCBs (plus at times, other stakeholders) will ensure that criteria for approval are clear, scientifically current, and well publicized and will help to promote consistency from one DCB to another for similar products.

The FDA as a Certifier of Certifiers

As well as addressing overarching safety concerns, the FDA will be responsible for certifying DCBs and signing off on marketing approvals. During the clinical testing and the DCB's evaluation of an NDA for a given product, the FDA will normally be exposed to the developing project to only a limited extent. Via periodic reports from the DCBs, the agency will receive information needed to monitor safety information, compile databases, and prepare to review the DCB's recommendations for drug approval. These reports will include a list of INDs issued (with the name of drug and sponsor), milestones (dates and numbers of patients in the various phases of clinical development), and ADEs. However, these communications shall not be used by the agency to create a more active role for itself in the oversight of clinical programs; most issues that arise in the course of drug development will be resolvable via sponsor-DCB interactions without involving the FDA. Although the FDA will not routinely have significant direct contact with the sponsor during the IND phase, the agency may, for cause, at any time inspect or audit the sponsor, DCB, or any other component of the drug development apparatus. An FDA inspection might be triggered, for example, by a suspected problem involving safety that has been inadequately addressed or information from a clinical investigator or institution that raises concerns about the integrity of data or the conduct of an investigator.

Once the NDA has been sent to the FDA with the DCB's recommendation for approval, the agency will have a fixed period—say, ninety days—to review the recommendation. During this period, the FDA commissioner will approve or, for a specified cause, reject the NDA (with an explanation that, in legal terms, must rebut the "rebuttable presumption" of the DCB's recommendation). The ninety-day period of review will not be extendable, and the commissioner's failure to act during this period will constitute assent to the drug's approval. If the FDA rejects the NDA, the DCB or the sponsor will be able to appeal the decision (a process that in turn must be completed in a further ninety days) via a mechanism that is described below.

Drug Certifying Bodies (DCBs)

Certification of DCBs by the FDA will ensure that they possess sufficient technical, scientific, and managerial expertise to oversee and review the testing of particular categories of products. This process of certification will be similar to, but more intensive than, the agency's current scrutiny of the qualifications of clinical investigators and institutions to perform clinical studies. It will be highly analogous to accreditation of third parties for the review of medical devices that now exists (see chapter 5). Certification could as well be modeled on the accreditation of nationally recognized testing laboratories by OSHA (see chapter 5) or on other analogous, complex health-related licensing procedures such as the Joint Commission on Accreditation of Healthcare Organizations (JCAHO).[8] The Joint Commission evaluates and accredits approximately 20,000 health care organizations in the United States, including hospitals, health care networks, managed care organizations, and other organizations that provide a wide spectrum of medical services.[9] It is

8. Miller and Wardell, "Therapeutic Drugs and Biologics," p. 49.
9. www.jcaho.org/who_we_are.html, accessed January 23, 2000.

not a government agency but an independent, not-for-profit organization.

Neither the FDA nor any other government agency will have a role
in determining other issues related to DCBs, such as their number,
corporate structure, or geographic distribution. A DCB could choose,
for example, to incorporate as a for-profit or not-for-profit organization.
It might choose to locate in existing centers of medical research or near
centers of the pharmaceutical or biotechnology industry. It might decide to specialize in particular therapeutic areas or drug types or to be
broadly qualified for a wide range of products. These issues will be
determined by the effects of market forces.

The Sponsor-DCB Relationship

A product sponsor will select a DCB from those certified for the appropriate product class—for example, psychotropics, antibiotics, metabo-
lism/endocrine, vaccines, and so on. The choice will be made in basi-
cally the same way all independent corporate decisions about hiring a
supplier or consultant are made. Critical to selection will be the perceived ability of the DCB to oversee a suitable preclinical and clinical
program and the likelihood of a timely review that will result in a
recommendation for approval and FDA concurrence. The nuances of
the agreement will reflect the particular needs of the sponsor and the
capabilities of the DCB. The level of service required will depend on
the client's preferences and on factors such as the size and previous
experience of the sponsor (both generally and for the particular class of
drug in question); the degree of novelty of the product; the presence of
particularly difficult issues of purity, potency, stability, or toxicity; and
the size and complexity of the clinical program. There will also be, on
occasion, other issues that require highly specialized experience in
public health and areas outside of medicine. In the case of influenza
vaccine, for example, appropriate formulation of the product and rapid
testing and approval would require consultation with public health
agencies about the appropriate viral strains to be included in the vac-

cine, in which case the sponsor might wish to select a DCB with expertise in this area. Sociological issues can also arise; for example, in the case of an HIV vaccine, it might be necessary to arrive at a consensus about what degree of efficacy—disease prevention—must be demonstrated to support licensure. This determination could be important in guarding against false assurances of immunity to infection that could convey the unintended implication that safe sex practices can be ignored. In such a situation, the sponsor might need to take the specialized experience of available DCBs into account.

As described above, the DCB retained by a drug sponsor will oversee most of the drug development process on a day-to-day basis. It will work with the sponsor during the preclinical phase and approve the commencement of clinical trials. Then, throughout the clinical testing, the DCB will ensure that the sponsor is in compliance with applicable regulatory standards including Good Laboratory Practices, Good Manufacturing Practices, and Good Clinical Practices, all of which are spelled out in current regulations and guidance documents. The DCB will be responsible for visiting and auditing the sponsor at specified junctures to ensure compliance. It will also be responsible for certifying that the original data are accurately recorded, analyzed, and reported; that the data are suitably archived for any necessary future audits; and that the summary analyses and reports accurately reflect the data. The criteria for approval of the NDA will remain those of the current law: safety and efficacy, as judged by experts. In this regulatory model, however, the frontline experts will be working for the DCB, not the government. As clinical testing is poised to begin, a second line of experts and safety overseers will be the research institutions' own institutional review boards (IRBs), which will provide independent affirmation of the appropriateness of the design of the trials, the informed consent, and other factors. These IRB panels, whose sole function is the protection of human research subjects, have scientific and lay members and already review all clinical protocols performed in research institutions. Arguably, IRBs alone could be entrusted with sole jurisdiction over phase I clinical trials, although that is not an element of this proposal.

The cooperative relationship between the DCB and client, and the DCB's close and continuous involvement with testing, will bring about a number of improvements to the system:

1. The DCB's early involvement with the sponsor will encourage the identification and solution of problems during the pre-IND submission period, so that there should be little delay once the IND is submitted.

2. The uncertainty surrounding arbitrary, unexpected regulatory obstacles early in clinical testing of a new product will be substantially reduced. Sponsors will no longer suffer the excessive risk averseness and intransigence toward phase I trials shown by the FDA—for example, permitting only single-dose, instead of dose-ranging, studies or requiring that trials begin at an inappropriately low dose, that unnecessary, invasive procedures be performed on patients, and even that foreign trials be completed and the results submitted before the U.S. trials can begin.

3. Because of its intense involvement, the DCB will often be able to begin work on the NDA review even as the data to support the application are still accumulating—a "developing" or "self-reviewing"[10] or "rolling" NDA[11]—which should reduce the length of time necessary to review a straightforward NDA from the 1999 FDA average of approximately a year and a half.

4. Even more important than shortening the NDA review period will be reducing the overall time of clinical testing—that is, from the filing of the IND to the approval of the NDA—which

10. Miller and Wardell, "Therapeutic Drugs and Biologics," p. 51.

11. Elaine M. Healy and Kenneth I. Kaitin, "The European Agency for the Evaluation of Medicinal Products' Centralized Procedure for Product Approval: Current Status," *Drug Information Journal* 33 (1999): 969–78.

has been increasing steadily for decades. Many potentially difficult issues to be addressed in the evaluation—such as mar-
ginal efficacy, low therapeutic index, and problems with safety,
stability, or manufacturing—will be identified and solved during the course of clinical testing under the IND.

5. The DCB will help the client to determine as early as possible
if and when development of a given product should be termi-
nated, a service that will avoid wasting precious investment
capital and one that the DCB will be better able to provide
than the more remote and less helpful FDA.

Overall, this new system will encourage an increasingly high level of
problem solving and efficiency, especially as the market learns to favor
those DCBs that maintain high standards and offer reliability, expeditiousness, and innovativeness.

The Appeals Process

Two factors have systematically discouraged industry from voicing com-
plaints about the content of FDA decisions or the agency's decision-
making process. First, there is a well-justified fear of agency reprisals;
FDA reviewers and managers have freely expressed their contempt
toward companies that question or complain about FDA decisions.
Even in the absence of serious, specific points of disagreement, the
atmosphere faced by industry is sometimes contentious. For example,
a director of the neuropharmacology division of the FDA's Center for
Drug Evaluation and Review (now retired) warned representatives of a
company at one point that he considered them "the enemy," that there
exists a fundamental conflict between the interests of industry and the
FDA, and that he intended to treat the company accordingly.[12]

Second (but not unrelated to the first), there has been no indepen-

12. Private communication from the CEO of a pharmaceutical company; name
withheld by request.

dent venue for appeals. At present, there is an FDA ombudsman with agencywide responsibilities, and there are ombudsmen at some of the agency's regulatory components, including the Center for Drug Evaluation and Review and Center for Biologics Evaluation and Review; but in general they are neither independent nor effective, nor are they highly regarded by industry. These ombudsmen all report to senior managers and are disinclined to make waves or to criticize their colleagues. A vigorous, independent agency ombudsman could help induce regulators to act in the public interest. However, the office would first have to be restructured to achieve the following: (1) independence from the agency and the FDA commissioner; (2) access to independent expertise in relevant disciplines, including medicine, pharmacology, science, regulation, and law; and (3) the power to levy sanctions against FDA employees found to be responsible, individually or collectively, for flawed decisions or policies that constitute severe, avoidable type 1 or type 2 errors. A strong agency ombudsman with these characteristics could offer a (partial) alternative to the more fundamental reform described in this volume.

In addition to ombudsmen, many FDA regulatory components have advisory committees (consisting largely of academic specialists) that offer a source of independent advice, but these committees have seldom been inclined to intervene on behalf of drug sponsors or to criticize agency policies; in recent years, they seem to have become even less independent of the agency. Their members are selected and managed by the FDA, and their chairmen often seem to be acting as agents of the agency. Moreover, the panels are frequently directed to address only narrow issues that are presented to them by FDA staff in a way that channels the experts in a preordained direction. Advisory committees are too often used to provide cover for unpopular or dubious decisions. Neither the existing ombudsmen nor the advisory committee system offers, therefore, the needed forum for assuring that FDA officials act expeditiously, fairly, impartially, and civilly.

The proposal described herein creates an appeal mechanism for DCB-FDA disagreements over product approval—an independent, standing advisory committee of experts, located organizationally in the Department of Health and Human Services (DHHS), where the FDA is located, at the level of the office of the secretary (therefore, not reporting to the FDA commissioner). The committee should be con-stituted of approximately ten to twenty distinguished, apolitical mem-bers representing patient groups, medical practitioners, medical scien-tists, and the drug industry. The membership of the committee will possess collectively a wide spectrum of scientific, medical, and regula-tory expertise and will be supplemented by the added expertise of ad hoc members when necessary. The committee will hear appeals of the FDA's rejections of a DCB recommendation and advise the secretary of DHHS, who, it is expected, will accept their advice and instruct the FDA commissioner to implement the committee's decision.

Reciprocity with Foreign Approvals

There has been gradual movement toward harmonization of various aspects of pharmaceutical oversight across national boundaries, includ-ing standardization of the format of submissions, the criteria for Good Clinical Practices, and mutual recognition of Good Manufacturing Practices inspections.[13] However, the FDA has refused to relinquish any of its perquisites or autonomy with respect to marketing approvals and has, therefore, resisted any suggestion of reciprocity on approvals. The agency's self-interested resistance notwithstanding, the high stan-dards and professionalism of oversight in the United Kingdom and in the supranational EMEA argue that at least certain foreign evaluations need not be completely duplicated in the United States. Therefore, the new system will permit the direct submission to the FDA of an approved registration package from the EMEA and certain foreign national reg-ulatory agencies, such as the U.K. Medicines Control Agency. These

---

13. Food and Drug Administration, Department of Health and Human Services, "International Conference on Harmonization. Good Clinical Practice: Consolidated Guideline; Notice of Availability," *Federal Register* 62 (May 9, 1997): 25691–709.

foreign agencies will be functionally equivalent to a domestic DCB in that they will submit to the FDA detailed summaries of the data on which a drug's approval was based, and the ninety-day time period for the FDA to review and approve or reject this package will apply. Alternatively, the sponsor of a drug that has obtained (or is en route to) foreign approval will be permitted to contract with a U.S. DCB to oversee its drug development regime and evaluate its NDA.

Status of the Current Regulations

This reform proposal conforms to the original intent of the existing statutes for drug development and approval—that is, to ensure the overall safety and effectiveness of drugs. The shift of even a significant proportion of regulatory responsibility to nongovernmental entities and experts will in no way compromise these goals. On the contrary, this revision will help to relieve the current distortion and overinterpretation of the statutes and to reverse the FDA's evolution far beyond what Congress could have foreseen. But even changes that fundamentally alter for the better regulators' incentives and disincentives, risks and rewards, will not be a panacea, and the system could benefit significantly from other reforms as well. Many of the FDA's existing regulations, regulatory interpretations, and policies, some of which have been discussed above, should be simplified and made more consistent with accepted medical practice, scientific principles, the intent of the law, and common sense. The FDA's willful interference with the promulgation to health professionals of peer-reviewed medical articles that discuss off-label uses is an affront to public health, and although the agency's intrusiveness has been partly remedied by the federal courts, FDA officials continue to try to circumvent the will of the judiciary (*vide supra*). Other worthy changes would include relegating the oversight of drugs' phase I trials exclusively to IRBs; wider use of accelerated approvals coupled with phase IV (that is, postmarketing) clinical studies; the introduction of automatic reciprocity in granting approvals between the United States and certain foreign regulatory agencies; and withdrawal of both the 1994 proposed regulation on the reporting of adverse drug experiences[14] and the 1998 regulation that requires increased drug testing in pediatric populations (see chapter 4).[15] It can also be argued that postmarketing surveillance of drugs needs improvement—perhaps even drastic revision—because neither the FDA nor the medical community currently has sufficient infrastructure to adequately detect, investigate, and prevent major adverse effects. Wood, Stein, and Woosley have proposed, for example, the creation of an independent drug safety board analogous to the National Transportation Safety Board, whose functions would be to "monitor drugs' safety, investigate reports of drug toxicity, and recommend actions to minimize the risks of drug therapy."[16]

Eventually, the new regulatory system envisioned here must be able to undertake such needed refinements, which may be in the direction of either greater or lesser control over the drug development process. It was only after careful consideration that I chose not to incorporate any such changes into this proposal because, although such adjustments would further improve drug regulation, they are not central to fundamental reform; and I wished not to distract attention from the more basic changes that characterize the proposal. Therefore, in order to provide for an orderly transition to the new system, maintain consistency with internationally harmonized formats, and avoid muddying the waters of regulatory reform by proposing too many changes simultaneously, the current regulations will initially be retained. As experience is gained with the new system during a transition period, a standing com-

---

14. Food and Drug Administration, Department of Health and Human Services, "Adverse Experience Reporting Requirements for Human Drug and Licensed Biological Products," *Federal Register* 59 (October 27, 1994): 54046–64.

15. Food and Drug Administration, Department of Health and Human Services, "Regulations Requiring Manufacturers to Assess the Safety and Effectiveness of New Drugs and Biological Products in Pediatric Patients," *Federal Register* 63 (1998): 66632–74.

16. Alastair J. J. Wood, C. Michael Stein, and Raymond Woosley, "Making Medicines Safer: The Need for an Independent Drug Safety Board," *New England Journal of Medicine* 339 (1998): 1851–54.

mittee made up of representatives from the FDA, drug sponsors, DCBs, patient groups, and academia will make recommendations for rule making to revise and simplify the regulations in order to improve the IND/NDA process within the constraints of the revised statute. This process might be conducted under the auspices of a nonideological expert group such as the Institute of Medicine.

To promote consistency in drug testing and review (which is now often lacking from division to division and even reviewer to reviewer at the FDA) from one DCB to another, up-to-date standards and guidance documents should be available. For example, it would be valuable for sponsors and DCBs to have "points to consider" documents that address technical issues as they arise, as well as updates on issues such as the standardization of formulations for human gene therapy and the appropriate uses of surrogate end points and placebo controls. These guidance documents should be produced jointly by the FDA, DCBs, and other stakeholders following a procedure to be determined. Two possible models for the production of such documents are already in place: the consensus-building conferences convened periodically by the National Institutes of Health and the process by which new product standards are developed by NRTLs for products within their purview (*vide supra*).

Other Related Reforms

Finally, although tort reform is beyond the scope of this proposal, remedies in this area are needed to remove the uncertainty and undue costs related to product liability, which, in combination with the excessive regulatory burden, threaten industrial innovation. Our litigious society and American companies' fear of lawsuits have negative consequences for both national competitiveness and public health. Viscusi has comprehensively reviewed the shortcomings of the current tort system and suggested remedies.[17] He is correct that there will be im-

17. W. Kip Viscusi, "Regulatory Reform and Liability for Pharmaceuticals and Medical Devices," in Epstein et al., *Advancing Medical Innovation*, pp. 79–102.

portant legal and practical consequences if nongovernmental certifiers or reviewers of drugs are exposed to significant potential liability; in other words, substantial and unpredictable liability will discourage potential new entrants into this market, and the desired competition among certifying organizations will not be forthcoming. Therefore, regulatory reform along the lines of that proposed in this volume should be accompanied by legislation that would recognize the validity of a regulatory compliance defense against litigation. Such a law would imply, in effect, that, when a pharmaceutical manufacturer meets the stringent and comprehensive regulatory requirements for product approval, any mishap from the product is wholly unforeseeable. It would stipulate, therefore, that manufacturers' liability is mitigated by the extensive regulatory control (by the FDA or an equivalent, as proposed herein) over their products from the earliest stages of clinical research to marketing approval, and over postmarket surveillance, the preparation of labeling, and advertising materials.[18] However, while Viscusi advocates that a regulatory compliance defense should be available to the DCBs for damages caused by unforeseen circumstances, he would not extend such protection for negligence. Such jeopardy would preserve certifiers' incentives to perform in a responsible and efficient manner, he concludes, while protecting them from liability for injuries or damages caused by a product that was developed, evaluated, and approved competently and in good faith. In addition, instead of joint-and-several liability, Viscusi suggests that there should be a system of proportionate liability that would hold a manufacturer liable only for the damage it actually causes, and that there be caps on noneconomic damages, such as pain and suffering.

18. Ibid.

Summary

Since the present system for the regulation of drugs in the United States was established in 1962, the monopolistic FDA has steadily increased the scope of its responsibilities and activities and, concomitantly, the regulatory burden on drug developers. The costs and time required for drug development have spiraled upward. The average time required to develop a drug has more than doubled, and the approximately half a billion dollars to bring a drug to market is by far the largest price tag anywhere in the world. During this time, ironically, fundamental changes have taken place in government, industry, medicine, and society that argue for a *less* costly, imperious, intrusive, and monopolistic system — one that will foster innovation without sacrificing safety. There is a broad consensus among those who study or interact with the FDA that the agency currently imposes more regulation of pharmaceuticals than is necessary and sufficient. Studies over more than forty years have repeatedly identified the same problems and suggested similar solutions. These remedies include broad, structural changes and specific improvements, all focused on reducing the time, cost, complexity, and unpredictability of the process. But the FDA has been slow and obdurate in implementing such changes, and Congress has not provided aggressive, effective oversight. The net effect has been a deterioration of the system and its ability to meet real public health needs.

Three things are clear: Reform of drug regulation is necessary, it must be fundamental in nature, and it must come from outside the agency via new legislation. The plan for reform proposed here maintains existing or equivalent standards—and assurance to consumers—of product purity, potency, and quality. It retains the legal requirement for premarket demonstration of new drugs' safety and effectiveness, the agency's final sign-off authority for product marketing, and the FDA's responsibility for overarching safety issues. The seminal change is that day-to-day oversight of drug testing and the initial NDA review will be performed by nongovernmental, FDA-certified entities: drug certifying bodies, or DCBs. The FDA thereby becomes primarily a *certifier of certifiers*, rather than a *certifier of products*. The proposed model (1) transfers much of the responsibility for oversight of clinical trials and NDA review to nongovernmental experts in the DCBs; (2) finances DCBs with user fees, via contractual arrangements between sponsors (drug manufacturers) and DCBs; (3) introduces competition among the DCBs for drug sponsor clients; and (4) also introduces competition between DCBs and certain foreign regulatory agencies that are certified to submit an approved registration package directly to the FDA.

Delegating a significant portion of the oversight responsibility to nongovernmental entities will simultaneously introduce into the regulation of drug development several positive elements: (1) competition among the DCBs for drug companies' business, creating pressure for greater innovativeness and efficiency in the oversight process; (2) competition between DCBs and the most respected European regulatory agencies (whose recommendation for approval would be tantamount to a positive recommendation from a U.S. DCB); and (3) a more appropriate balance than presently exists between regulators' own incentives and disincentives, risks and rewards. This potent combination of competition and incentives to become more efficient at getting safe, effective drugs to patients can transform the drug development process and reverse the current upward spiral of increasing time and costs. The public will benefit directly by earlier access to greater numbers of less costly drugs, and indirectly by greater robustness and productivity in the pharmaceutical industry.

Index